Praise for The Vegetarian Solution

"The medical research documenting the power of a vegetarian diet, composed of whole grains, fruits, vegetables and legumes, to improve our health is compelling. This research shows that a vegetarian diet can help prevent, and in many cases even reverse, many of the common diseases that we suffer from today. The Vegetarian Solution *makes the latest research, on the benefits of a vegetarian diet for our health and the world we live in, easy to understand and contains many practical points of information. I highly recommend* The Vegetarian Solution *to all those wanting to maintain or regain their health."*

—Neal Barnard, M.D.
President, Physicians Committee for Responsible Medicine

*"*The Vegetarian Solution *is a factual, scientific-literature-supported treatment of a most important subject. The upbeat and fun-filled perspective is refreshing and makes the facts actually most interesting and easy to read. The wide ranging subjects that impinge on vegetarianism and vegetarians are very broad and treated with respect and admiration in Stewart Rose's book.*

The fact is, that reading this book and being motivated and making changes in your eating habits, has the potential of adding years to your life and life to your years. It is your life and you are what you eat!"

—Ray Foster, M.D., F.A.C.S.
Staff Physician, Black Hills Health and Education Center

*"*The Vegetarian Solution *is power-packed with scientific support for vegetarian nutrition, and practical pointers on how to adopt this type of diet. In addition, the writing style is lively and easy to understand. This will be a good reference source for many years to come – one that I will strongly recommend to patients, friends and relatives."*

—F. Patricia McEachrane-Gross, M.D., M.P.H.
Chief, Department of Medical Management
OIC, Medical Evaluation Board Process
USA MEDDAC

"For those seeking to make kinder food choices for animals, the environment and themselves, The Vegetarian Solution *offers simple and understandable ways to make the switch to a vegetarian lifestyle."*

—Annette Laico
Executive Director, Progressive Animal Welfare Society (PAWS)

D1362013

"The Vegetarian Solution *presents the most comprehensive evidence in favor of a vegetarian diet I have ever read. It is solidly referenced to convince even the most scholarly health professional, and yet practical and easy to understand for the average lay person.*

From heart disease to hemorrhoids and fossil fuels to faith, Stewart Rose does so much more than merely saying vegetarianism "is healthier for you." The facts are researched and the illustrations are drawn from every conceivable angle to build a most comprehensive argument that not only are you *what you eat but so is the world."*

— **Timothy Riesenberger, M.D., M.P.H.**
West Sound Emergency Physicians

"As health care costs escalate and our resources are stretched to the breaking point, is there only inevitable disaster ahead of us? Are we doomed to die from diabetes, heart disease, cancer or other chronic diseases? Will we be overwhelmed by famine, world wide hunger and global warming? Is there no hope for our planet? Stewart Rose has done a superb job in gathering the facts documenting The Vegetarian Solution. *Well referenced and yet easy to read, this is a must read book for anyone interested in health or the welfare of our planet."*

— **Keith Hanson, M.D.**
Chief of Staff, Okanogan-Douglas District Hospital
Medical Director, Coronary Health Improvement Program,
Brewster, Washington

"It is increasingly clear that eating the right diet can help to prevent many of the major diseases that afflict us and can help to combat these diseases once they have begun. Switching to a whole plant food [vegetarian] diet is perhaps the single most important choice most people can ever make for achieving good health and avoiding disease. This book is a helpful introduction to the health benefits of a vegetarian diet."

— **Michael J. Orlich, M.D.**
Academic Dean, Weimar College
Physician, NEWSTART Lifestyle Program

"Stewart Rose is a scholar and ambassador for the ages-old philosophy and practice of abstaining from animal flesh. He emphasizes the rewards of vegetarianism: people return to their natural, health-supporting diet, animals are spared the slaughterhouse, and the Earth's vast resources are more efficiently used. To live upon the foods of the plant kingdom is logical, civilized, and can bring forth the higher thoughts and feelings within man and woman. Stewart Rose is a grassroots leader of the 21st Century American Vegetarian Movement – and the grassroots is where it began. This book inspires and guides others on the local level to continue or initiate work for the great cause."

— **Karen Iacobbo and Michael Iacobbo**
Authors, *Vegetarians and Vegans in America Today,* and
Vegetarian America: A History

*Improve Your Health
and the World You Live In*

The Vegetarian Solution

YOUR ANSWER TO CANCER, HEART DISEASE, GLOBAL WARMING, AND MORE

Stewart Rose

Healthy Living Publications
Summertown, Tennessee

9-26-8

Senior Editor: *Amanda Strombom*
Managing Editor: *Griggs Irving*
Copy Editors: *Michael M. Angulo and Jo Stepaniak*
Cover Design: *Aerocraft Charter Art Service*
Interior Design: *Edwina Cusolito*
Illustrations: *Casey McDonald and Jessica Dadds*

Healthy Living Publications
a division of Book Publishing Company
PO Box 99
Summertown, TN 38483
1-888-260-8458
www.bookpubco.com

Printed in Canada.

ISBN 978-1-57067-205-7

17 16 15 14 13 12 11 10 09 08 07   9 8 7 6 5 4 3 2 1

The Book Publishing Co. is a member of Green Press Initiative. We have elected to print this title on paper with postconsumer recycled content and processed chlorine free, which saved the following natural resources:

26 trees
1,236 lbs of solid waste
9,625 gallons of water
2,319 lbs of greenhouse gases
18 million BTUs

For more information visit: www.greenpressinitiative.org. Savings calculations thanks to the Environmental Defense Paper Calculator at www.papercalculator.org

Library of Congress Cataloging-in-Publication Data

Rose, Stewart D., 1956-
The vegetarian solution : your answer to cancer, heart disease, global warming and more / by Stewart D. Rose.
    p. cm.
  Includes bibliographical references and index.
  ISBN 978-1-57067-205-7
  1. Vegetarianism. I. Title.

  RM236.R67 2007
  613.2'62--dc22
              2007001136

The information in this book is for educational purposes only. The information is not intended as a substitute for a physician's diagnosis and care. The author urges everyone, including those with medical problems or symptoms, to consult a licensed physician before undertaking any lifestyle or medical changes.

Contents

(Continued)

*For my dear wife, Susan, whose love is the
foundation of my life.*

*For my teacher Mr. Rotenberg,
who wouldn't start a class each day until every
student performed an act of charity.*

For the six million—may I be worthy of them.

Acknowledgements

I'd like to thank the President of Vegetarians of Washington, Amanda Strombom, for her editing and considerable contribution to the book. She spent many hours working through the key points of the text. Amanda has worked hard to build a vegetarian society strong enough to support the writing of its third book. Griggs Irving, managing editor of the Vegetarians of Washington book team, has been a driving force towards completion of this book. Were it not for the combination of wisdom and perseverance that Griggs brings to every project, this book might never have been completed. I would also like to thank Edwina Cusolito for crafting and designing the layout of the book. Edwina's heart is matched only by her patience. Thanks also go to Michael M. Angulo for stepping in to copy edit for this inexperienced author, and to Jessica Dadds and Casey McDonald for creating the illustrations and tables that add so much to this book. I would also like to thank Tim Fargo and Anne I. Johnson for their article "The Environmental Case for Vegetarianism," which appeared in our first book, *Veg-Feasting in the Pacific Northwest,* and for teaching me so much about the connection between our food choices and the environment we live in. I'd like to thank Cheryl Redmond for her article "The Vegetarian Kitchen," which first appeared in *The Veg-Feasting Cookbook.* This article was very helpful to me in my research for Chapter 2 of this book. I am also grateful to the many members, volunteers, and supporters of Vegetarians of Washington, too many to mention individually, for their continued dedication and support. One could not hope for a better publisher than the Book Publishing Company. I thank Bob and Cynthia Holzapfel and everyone on the Book Publishing Company team for contributing so much wise guidance to this project.

Preface

This book is based upon the many classes and speeches I have given as vice-president of Vegetarians of Washington, and the many requests for more detailed information in printed form. The topics covered include the ones most commonly requested by our members. Also included is information that many of the members feel is not readily available elsewhere.

The list of benefits of a vegetarian diet is very long indeed. Many people have requested a book that covers the subject broadly but not superficially. There is a call for a book that has solid information but doesn't require special training and knowledge to read and appreciate it.

I want to provide health-related information of concern to as wide a cross-section of people as possible. For instance, many moms and pregnant women have approached me over the years with requests for information addressing their special concerns. Many teens and seniors also have questions and specific issues of concern to them.

I feel there is a need for a book that presents the clear benefits that following a vegetarian diet has for the environment and the problem of global hunger. There is also a demand for a book that surveys various cultural and spiritual issues. Many people want to know how following a vegetarian diet will fit in with their daily lives. Too many people think that it is somehow complicated or difficult to follow a vegetarian diet. With this book, I want to show them just how easy and delicious a vegetarian diet really is.

Finally, I feel that it is very important to show that the eight million vegetarians in the country today are made up of a diverse assortment of everyday people, who form a microcosm of the American people as a whole, and that many of our country's and the world's greatest historical figures have advocated and followed a vegetarian diet.

This book will have achieved these goals if it helps the reader to understand the profound power our food choices have on our health and the world we live in.

Stewart Rose, *Vice President*
Vegetarians of Washington

Chapter 1

Introduction

The food we choose to eat is usually the single most important determinant of our health and longevity. Modern medical studies show again and again that a vegetarian diet is the best way to reduce our risk of many of the common diseases currently plaguing our society, such as heart disease, cancer, and diabetes. It also forms a very valuable part of the treatment of these diseases.

When it comes to a healthful diet, many people mistakenly believe they are caught in a bind between wholesome food and great taste. A vegetarian diet supplies the perfect solution to this dilemma by offering the most delicious-tasting food imaginable while providing the highest-quality nutrition available.

But a vegetarian diet is not just a solution to our health problems. According to the United Nations Food and Agriculture Organization, livestock and meat production contribute more to global warming than all the cars, buses, trains, planes, and ships put together. Livestock rearing is also the main cause of rainforest destruction, and runoff from this industry is the cause of much of the water pollution the world over. There's a good feeling that comes from helping to sustain our land, air, and water. A vegetarian diet provides a very powerful solution to the environmental crisis we currently face.

Most of today's meat comes from factory farms, a perversion of traditional farming. These farms are designed to produce meat efficiently and cheaply. The problem is that the modern factory farm and slaughterhouse have created conditions that are very harsh for the farm animals. A vegetarian diet provides a solution to the feeling we have in the back of our minds whenever we stop to ponder just how that hamburger arrived on our plate.

The problem of global hunger is staggering in both its scope and consequences. Using staple crops to feed farm animals is very wasteful. Most of the nutrition, in some cases as much 90 percent, is lost by the time it gets to us in the form of meat. The largest food reserve in the world is the food we waste by feeding it to animals. In many ways, a vegetarian diet forms an essential part of the solution to the problem of global hunger. If the land used to grow animal feed were instead used to grow crops for the world's hungry, there could be enough for all. A vegetarian meal can be an act of charity for those in need.

The food we bless at the dinner table has always been a primary concern of every faith and tradition. Many people are pleasantly surprised to learn of the support all the major religions voice for a vegetarian diet. They also appreciate knowing that many widely respected religious leaders have been vegetarian or have advocated the desirability of a vegetarian diet. Many people find that a vegetarian diet supplies a spiritually satisfying solution to the religious mandates of all major faiths to preserve health and honor Creation.

So just who are the vegetarians and where are they to be found? The big news is that vegetarians are everywhere these days, and in fact, they always have been an important part of our society. They have made contributions

Defining Vegetarian

The word "vegetarian" is generally thought to refer to a diet that excludes all meat, poultry, and fish products. However, there are various subsets of this. A lacto-ovo vegetarian diet excludes meat, poultry, and fish products but includes eggs and dairy. An ovo-vegetarian diet includes eggs but not dairy. Similarly, a lacto-vegetarian diet includes dairy but not eggs. A total vegetarian diet, often called a vegan diet includes all plant foods but excludes meat, poultry, fish, dairy, and eggs.

The original goal of a vegetarian diet was to promote our health and well-being, while showing mercy and compassion for farm animals. Recent information about the saturated fat and cholesterol found in eggs and dairy, and the impact of modern methods of egg and dairy production on animal welfare, would seem to necessitate refining what we mean by "vegetarian" in order to stay in line with its original intent.

Therefore, I define "vegetarian" as a diet that excludes all meat, poultry, fish, dairy, and eggs. Where scientific studies use the term "vegetarian" to mean lacto-ovo vegetarian, I have tried to make this clear, but this difference in terminology should be remembered when reading any referenced studies.

in all walks of life throughout history. Examples include Albert Einstein in science, Thomas Edison in industry, Olympic gold medalist Carl Lewis, rock star Paul McCartney of the Beatles, and founding father Benjamin Franklin, to name just a few. But most vegetarians are not famous. They're the people who live next door, the lady who sits next to you at work, and the guy standing behind you in line at the movies. They're everyday people making a wise and delicious choice.

Switching over to a vegetarian diet, or even just including more vegetarian foods in your meal, is an adventure that is both interesting and fun. Trying new foods and learning as you go will give you a chance to be creative. The secrets of success on your journey are to be willing to learn about and experiment with new foods, to proceed at your own pace, and just to do the best you can. Take the optimistic approach. However far you come on your journey will put you that much further ahead.

In this book, you will find much information about the many benefits of a vegetarian diet. Some reasons for moving toward a vegetarian diet will appeal to you more than others. Many people often change to a vegetarian diet for one reason, only to discover many other benefits to changing their diets which they hadn't before realized. So bear this in mind as you read this book, be open-minded about all the different benefits of a vegetarian diet, and pretty soon you'll be wondering what you were waiting for.

It's Natural

Many people think that humans are omnivores, meant to eat both meat and plant foods, and that a vegetarian diet is not natural. The fact is that nothing could be further from the truth. Humans are natural herbivores. This position is not "alternative" science; it's hardcore, mainstream, scientific thought. This is affirmed by Dr. William Clifford Roberts, editor in chief of the *American Journal of Cardiology,* who states, "Although we think we are one and we act as if we are one, human beings are not natural carnivores.... Flesh was never intended for human beings who are natural herbivores."

All animals can be classified into three groups according to their diets. Carnivores are meat eaters, omnivores eat both meat and vegetation, and herbivores eat only fruits, grains, vegetables, nuts, and legumes.

Anatomy and Physiology Comparisons (Table 1.1)

Carnivores

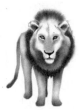

Incisor Teeth: Short pointed
Molar Teeth: Sharp
Nails: Sharp claws
Saliva: No digestive enzymes
Stomach Acid: pH of 1 with food in stomach
Small Intestine: 3–6 times body length
Urine: Extremely concentrated
Perspires Through Skin Pores: No

Omnivores

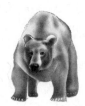

Incisor Teeth: Short pointed
Molar Teeth: Sharp
Nails: Sharp claws
Saliva: No digestive enzymes
Stomach Acid: pH of 1 with food in stomach
Small Intestine: 4–6 times body length
Urine: Extremely concentrated
Perspires Through Skin Pores: No

Herbivores

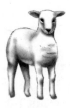

Incisor Teeth: Broad and flattened
Molar Teeth: Flattened
Nails: Flattened nails, hooves
Saliva: Carbohydrate digesting enzymes
Stomach Acid: pH of 4–5 with food in stomach
Small Intestine: 10–12 times body length
Urine: Moderately concentrated
Perspires Through Skin Pores: Yes

Humans

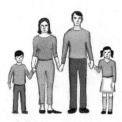

Incisor Teeth: Broad and flattened
Molar Teeth: Flattened
Nails: Flattened nails
Saliva: Carbohydrate digesting enzymes
Stomach Acid: pH of 4–5 with food in stomach
Small Intestine: 10–11 times body length
Urine: Moderately concentrated
Perspires Through Skin Pores: Yes

As can be seen in Table 1.1, the anatomy and physiology of humans closely match those of an herbivore—far more closely than they do to those of a carnivore or an omnivore.

A classical example of an omnivore is the dog. When dogs have huge amounts of saturated fat and cholesterol added to their diets, no damage to their arteries results. In fact, it is virtually impossible to produce atherosclerosis (clogging of the arteries) in dogs. This is true even when they consume an amount of saturated fat and cholesterol equal to a hundred times what an adult man would ordinarily consume in the typical American diet. On the other hand, adding as little as two grams of cholesterol to a rabbit's diet produces atherosclerotic changes in only two months. Dr. William S. Collins, professor of clinical medicine at Downstate Medical Center in New York City, concludes that man is vegetarian by design.

Ask yourself this question: Can you or anyone you know chase down a zebra, kill it with your bare hands, and then cut through its hide with your fingernails and teeth? Now ask yourself if there is anyone you know who can't peel a banana.

We can only eat animals through the use of tools and technology. While our growing brains have allowed for the increasing use of this technology over time, our bodies have remained unchanged. We can go against our nature for a while, but sooner or later an unnatural diet will catch up with us. And when it does, disease is the result. It would have been truly unfair for us to have been designed to eat meat only to acquire so many diseases from eating meat.

It may take a while to get used to the idea that a vegetarian diet is natural and that eating meat is the alternative. Maybe this will help. It may interest you to know that Charles Darwin was a vegetarian. Need someone more contemporary? OK. Did you know that the world-famous anthropologist Jane Goodall is a vegetarian?

Why not consider a switch to a vegetarian diet? After all, it's only natural!

It's Healthful

Who wouldn't want to live a longer and healthier life? While many people search the world over for the fountain of youth, the answer lies closer to home—in your own kitchen! There is no diet more nutritious than a vegetarian diet. The standard food groups typically include dairy products, eggs, meat, fish, and chicken. The new vegetarian food groups are fruits, vegetables, grains, legumes, and nuts.

As you will learn in this book, people who follow a vegetarian diet have much lower rates of many common diseases, including heart disease, hypertension (high blood pressure), stroke, cancer, and diabetes, just to name a few. Advantages are seen at all ages and for all demographic groups. Vegetarian children have a much lower rate of several childhood cancers; women have lower rates of diseases such as osteoporosis; men have lower rates of prostate cancer; seniors have lower rates of Parkinson's disease and dementia. The list goes on and on.

A vegetarian diet helps prevent many diseases. But what about those who are already suffering from a disease? Several studies show that a vegetarian diet will also help many of these patients get well again.

Let's take a look at atherosclerosis, clogged arteries that can lead to a heart attack. Texas cardiologist Dean Ornish became world famous for proving that a low-fat vegetarian diet would unclog his patients' arteries in just a few months. More recent studies show that a healthy vegetarian diet will lower patients' cholesterol levels more than the leading drug used to treat this condition, and it will do so without any side effects!

The proof is in the living. Several studies show that vegetarians live longer than those who eat the standard American diet. In fact, vegetarians who live in Loma Linda, California, the town with the highest proportion of vegetarians in America, have the longest life spans in the country. The men in this community live an average of nine and a half years longer and women an average of six years longer than the average American. In fact, according to Dr. Joel Fuhrman, author of *Eat to Live,* it might even be longer. He states, "Those who lived longest were those following the vegetarian diet the longest, and when we look at the subset who had followed a vegetarian diet for at least half their life, it appears they lived about 13 years longer." Think about it. That's a serious amount of time. It's not just in California either. Studies done in several other countries also show a longer and healthier life span for vegetarians.

What did these people have to do to live longer and healthier lives? All they had to do was to enjoy one delicious vegetarian meal after the other. In fact, the single most important thing your doctor could recommend to you that would have the greatest impact on your life would be to follow a vegetarian diet consisting of fruits, vegetables, grains, nuts, and legumes.

It's Easy

Perhaps you think following a vegetarian diet is complicated. Maybe you think you couldn't get enough protein. If you have a busy lifestyle, maybe you think you will have to give up convenience foods if you go vegetarian. Some people worry that they'll only be able to find the ingredients they need at an obscure store in the foothills of the Himalayas. Others worry that following a diet that will save their heart and colon will cost them an arm and a leg.

Well, worry no more. Following a vegetarian diet couldn't be easier or more delicious. All you need to get started is a good cookbook and the willingness to embark on an adventure in good eating.

Are you wondering what there is to buy? Recent years have seen a veritable explosion in the vegetarian food industry. Even your local supermarket is likely to carry veggie burgers and soymilk. Specialty stores and natural food markets now abound with a variety of vegetarian food. In fact, natural food stores are springing up all over the country to meet the demand of people looking for healthier options.

Are you too busy to cook? No need to worry! You can buy ready-to-microwave dishes such as tofu lasagne, soy dogs to take to the ball game, or a heat-and-serve Indian vegetable curry ... yum! Going out to eat has also never been easier, as the number of vegetarian and veg-friendly restaurants continues to increase. Even most conventional restaurants now carry vegetarian options.

Are you frightened by the prospect of counting grams of protein? Put away your calculator. Protein is abundantly available in plant foods, as Table 1.2 shows. The Food and Nutrition Board of the National Research Council states that you need 8–10 percent of your calories from protein. As you can see, if you eat sufficient calories and a variety of nutritious foods, you will find that it is impossible not to get enough protein.

In fact, protein deficiency is virtually unknown in the developed world, and many modern diseases are caused by an excess, rather than a lack, of protein in the diet.

The idea of combining proteins, such as having beans with rice, started back in the sixties with a book called *Diet for a Small Planet*. However, modern science has shown conclusively that protein combining is completely unnecessary, and even the author of that book, now older and wiser, acknowledges that her original conclusions were misleading. Our bodies keep a reservoir of amino acids (the building blocks of proteins) and draw from

It's Easy to Get the Protein You Need From Plant
Foods (Table 1.2)

Protein is shown as a percentage of calories

Vegetables	Protein	Legumes & Grains	Protein
Spinach	49%	Lentils	29%
Broccoli	45%	Pinto beans	26%
Kale	45%	Chickpeas	23%
Mushroom	39%	Peanuts	18%
Okra	27%	Sunflower seeds	17%
Tomato	20%	Wheat	17%
Pumpkin	15%	Oatmeal–cooked	15%
Corn	15%	Cashews	12%
Potato	11%	Rice–brown	8%

*Akers Keith, "A Vegetarian Source Book," Vegetarian Press,
Denver Colorado, 1989*

this reserve as needed. As long as you have a reasonably varied diet over the course of several days, you'll do fine. In fact, you'll do better than just fine. There's a reason vegetarians on average live much longer than others.

Are you watching your budget? Being a vegetarian shouldn't cost any more than the diet you're following now. And while you won't be spending any more money at the market or at a restaurant, you'll most likely be saving plenty of money at the doctor's office. In fact, the health care costs directly attributable to meat consumption amount to more than $60 billion annually.

There's a simple formula for easy shopping, delicious meals, and good health. Just remember to eat plenty of fruits, vegetables, grains, nuts, and legumes.

It's Tasty

Food provides pleasure as well as sustenance. Does it taste good? is the question that precedes every bite we put in our mouths. Our tongues signal the flavor and our mouths sense the texture.

Raw, steamed, or roasted vegetables, whole or ground nuts, steamed or toasted grains, chopped or sliced fruit, and baked or boiled beans all create a vast range of delicious tastes and textures. Serve any of these with rice, noodles, or potatoes, add some textural products such as tofu, tempeh, or seitan, and season with a splash of soy sauce or hot pepper sauce and a sprinkle of salt and herbs. Finish your meal with fresh fruit or frozen soy or rice "ice cream" covered with fruit or chocolate sauce.

Make a casserole, barbecue on the grill, blend, fry, bake, or steam—there are so many flavorful ways to combine, cook, and present vegetarian foods. A vegetarian diet presents you with such a delicious diversity of dishes to enjoy, whether home-cooked or in a restaurant.

Travel the world through your meals, from Mediterranean falafel to Mexican burritos, from Indian curries to Italian pasta dishes, from Szechwan noodles with stir-fried vegetables to Japanese vegetable sushi, from the finest gourmet restaurants in Paris to the ancient and delicate flavors of Persia. Stop in Thailand, as you savor exotic spices with each bite of scrumptious Thai food. After enjoying the finest cuisine the world has to offer, return to North America, where a vegetarian Thanksgiving will really stick to your ribs.

Vegetarian food is so good that it will grab you by the taste buds and it won't let go. Each meal you have will be made even more enjoyable by the realization that you'll finish it even healthier than when you began.

It's Popular

Who are vegetarians anyway? The answer may surprise you.

If you choose to follow a vegetarian diet, you'll be traveling in very distinguished company. Take a look on page 20 for a list of some famous vegetarians in history. You'll find both scientific and creative geniuses, great statesman and civic leaders, artists, actors, and superstar athletes.

Consider just a brief list of vegetarians who contributed so much. Leonardo da Vinci, Charles Darwin, Sir Isaac Newton, and Albert Einstein all accomplished their works of genius while following a vegetarian diet. Founding father Benjamin Franklin led America to freedom on a vegetarian diet. Creative inventors such as Thomas Edison and gifted musicians such as Gustav Mahler gave the world lasting treasures while following a vegetarian diet. Courageous women such as Clara Barton, who founded the American Red Cross, and Susan B. Anthony, who lead the movement to give women the right to vote, achieved all that they did on a vegetarian diet. In athletics,

Famous Vegetarians (Table 1.3)

Men and Women in American History

Susan B. Anthony, Women's Suffrage

Clara Barton, founder of American Red Cross

Benjamin Franklin, founding father

Sylvester Graham, creator of the Graham cracker

Thomas Jefferson (near vegetarian)

Coretta Scott King, wife of Dr. Martin Luther King, Jr.

Doctors

Henry Heimlich, M.D.

John Harvey Kellogg, M.D.

Dean Ornish, M.D.

Albert Schweitzer, M.D.

Benjamin Spock, M.D

Scientists

Charles Darwin

Leonardo DaVinci

Albert Einstein

Jane Goodall

Isaac Newton

Religious Leaders

General William Booth, founder of Salvation Army

His Holiness the Dalai Lama

Mahatma Ghandi

Abraham Kook, First Chief Rabbi Israel

John Wesley, founder of Methodist church

Ellen G. White, a founder of the Seventh Day Adventist church

Philosophers

Confucius

Plato

Pythagoras

Socrates

Industry

Thomas Edison, inventor of the light bulb

Steve Jobs, founder of Apple Computers

Isaac Pitman, inventor of shorthand

Military

Hugh Dowding, Air Chief Marshall Battle of Britain

Sports

Hank Aaron, Homerun record holder

Desmond Howard, Super Bowl MVP

Scott Jurek, Ultra-Marathon Champion

Carl Lewis, Track & field winner of nine Olympic Gold medals

Martina Navratilova, Tennis star

Bill Pearl, four-time Mr. Universe

Dave Scott, six-time triathlon winner

Music

Maxine Andrews, the Andrews Sisters

John William Coltrane

Skeeter Davis

Gustav Holst

Gustav Mahler

Paul McCartney

Olivia Newton John

Shania Twain

Eddie Veder, Pearl Jam

Moby

Hollywood

Bob Barker

James Cromwell

Cameron Diaz

Clint Eastwood

Dustin Hoffman

Toby McGuire

Natalie Portman

William Shatner

Alicia Silverstone

Mary Tyler Moore

Authors and Playwrights

Louisa May Alcott

George Bernard Shaw

Percy Shelley

Robert Louis Stevenson

Henry David Thoreau

Leo Tolstoy

H.G. Wells

Carl Lewis won nine Olympic gold medals and Bill Pearl was named Mr. America and Mr. Universe while performing on vegetarian fuel.

Growing in popularity, vegetarianism has now gone mainstream. Polls show that there are now about eight million Americans following a vegetarian diet. Also growing in popularity are the dishes produced by the many new vegetarian food companies and restaurants. In fact, vegetarian is America's trendiest cuisine, attracting the most gifted and creative chefs. Even the finest cooking schools in France now feature training in vegetarian cuisine.

From high school and college students to baby boomers and senior citizens, everyone seems to be discovering the many and the oh-so-delicious advantages of a vegetarian diet. Today, you'll find vegetarian meals offered just about everywhere. You'll find them in many schools, hospitals, and some fire stations. Even federal prisons now offer vegetarian meals. It's all the rage!

In this book you'll learn what it is about following a vegetarian diet that's exciting such a wide range of people. First, you'll see how easy it is to follow a vegetarian diet. You'll get to know what we call the "new food groups"—our simple way of ensuring that you get all the nutrition you need. You'll discover the best places to shop and eat out, and what to do when you're invited to other people's homes.

You'll learn about the many profound health advantages of a vegetarian diet. There's a reason that, on average, vegetarians live several years longer than others. You'll see how a health-promoting vegetarian diet not only helps to prevent a wide range of diseases but also helps those already suffering from disease to get well again. You'll discover how a vegetarian diet helps protect the environment. Sustainability is a key concept for today's world, and a vegetarian diet helps reduce both air and water pollution and helps to save the rainforests. Perhaps most important of all, the production of vegetarian food is far more efficient than raising cattle, and can make more food available to feed the world's hungry.

Today's farms are designed to run very differently than in the past. Conditions are much harsher for animals than they used to be. You'll soon see that following a vegetarian diet is not only good for your health, it really makes a difference to our animal friends as well.

Finally, we'll take a survey of the world religions. You'll be surprised to learn that a vegetarian diet has the support of many of the world's religious and spiritual leaders, past and present.

Chapter 2

Moving Toward a Vegetarian Diet

In this chapter you will get lots of tips for changing your diet. You'll take a look at the new food groups and see how to incorporate them into your daily life.

The New Food Groups

Everyone from medical researchers to family doctors is recommending a vegetarian diet these days. One report after another describes how vegetarians live longer and have much lower rates of heart disease, cancer, diabetes, and many other diseases. But just how do they do it? Do they walk through the market with charts and calculators following some complicated formula? What's their secret?

Well, there is no secret, and it's as easy as can be. Vegetarians simply include legumes, nuts and seeds, whole grains, vegetables, and fruits in their diets every day. By choosing a variety of foods from these five food groups, vegetarians have easily become the healthiest people in town. And the best part of it all is that vegetarian food is so delicious.

Let's take a closer look at what's included in each of the new food groups.

Legumes

Legumes include peas, lentils, and all kinds of beans: soybeans, chickpeas (also known as garbanzos), kidney beans, black beans, white beans, and even peanuts. All are packed with protein, complex carbohydrates including lots of fiber, calcium, and iron. They have no cholesterol and make a great replacement for meat in your diet.

Products made from soybeans, such as tofu and tempeh, offer a convenient way to include more soy in your diet. These foods are extremely versatile, absorbing the flavors of the cooking sauce you use, so they make effective

The New Food Groups (Table 2.1)
Dish these up for a healthy diet

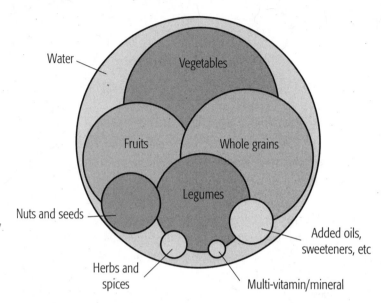

substitutes for meat in many traditional dishes such as Sloppy Joes, chili, or curries. Many of today's commercial meat substitutes are based on soy, such as veggie burgers, meatless hot dogs, and soy jerky, bacon, pepperoni, and bologna. Dairy alternatives, such as soymilk, soy cheese, soy yogurt, and soy ice cream, have also become very popular and are much more health-promoting than their dairy equivalents.

Nuts and Seeds

High in protein, nuts and seeds are also an excellent source of vitamins, minerals, fiber, "good" fats, and essential fatty acids (EFAs). (EFAs are fatty acids that are required in the human diet, but they must be obtained from food, as the body has no way of producing them internally). Include a handful of walnuts, cashews, almonds, Brazil nuts, or hazelnuts in your diet several times a week, or try nut butters for spreads, dips, and sauces. Pumpkin seeds, sesame seeds, and sunflower seeds add nutrients and crunch to your diet. Tahini, a spread made from ground sesame seeds, is one of the key ingredients in hummus, which is a great dip for vegetables.

Components of a Healthful Diet (Table 2.2)

Food	Recommended Amount	Common Examples
Legumes	Several servings each day	Soy, lentils, all kinds of beans, peas, peanuts, served as tofu, tempeh, curries, stews, soy milk etc.
Nuts and Seeds	A handful several times a week	Almonds, walnuts, cashews, sunflower seeds, sesame seeds, served raw, toasted or as nut milks and butters.
Whole Grains	Several servings each day	Wheat, oats, barley, rice served as bread, grains, pasta, cereals and some baked goods
Vegetables	Several servings each day	Broccoli, kale, spinach, carrots, tomatoes, eggplant, and sweet potatoes served fresh or cooked.
Fruit	Several servings each day	Oranges, apples, bananas, blueberries, melon, grapes, dates, served fresh, dried or as juices or smoothies
Herbs and Spices	Use generously to flavor your food	Garlic, onions, chili powder, curry, basil, oregano, cilantro
Vegetable Oils, Vinegars, Sweeteners and Treats	Use moderately	Olive oil, canola oil, balsamic vinegar, rice vinegar, maple syrup, black-strap molasses, dark chocolate
Water	6-8 cups a day	Teas, juices and water
Multi-vitamin	One a day	Make sure it includes B-12

Whole Grains

Whole grains include wheat, oats, barley, buckwheat, brown rice, cereals, pasta, and whole grain breads of every kind. Also included are less familiar grains such as quinoa and amaranth, which are quickly increasing in popularity. Whole grains are powerhouses of energy and nutrition, with generous amounts of protein, B vitamins and vitamin E, minerals such as iron and zinc, and fiber. There's an endless variety of ways to include whole grains in your diet. Try whole wheat toast or oatmeal for breakfast, a whole grain burrito or pasta for lunch, and brown rice or quinoa with your dinner. Everyone needs treats once in a while, so instead of more refined ingredients, use whole grain flour and natural sweeteners, such as maple syrup, brown rice syrup, or molasses to make tasty cakes and cookies.

Vegetables

The range of vegetables available is amazing, and every one of them is packed with vitamins, minerals, and fiber, plus an abundance of phytochemicals (compounds found only in plants and that have a beneficial effect on health). The cruciferous vegetables, broccoli, cauliflower, cabbage, kale, and collard greens, are especially well regarded both for their nutritional content and their ability to protect against disease. Green leafy vegetables, such as chard, spinach, arugula, and the many varieties of lettuce, provide excellent nutrition in salads. Tomatoes and peppers (both of which are technically fruits) are tasty in salads and sauces and are high in vitamins and antioxidants. Eggplants and potatoes make great foundations for any meal. Versatile vegetables can be served as side dishes or as a main dish and can be steamed, baked, or stir-fried.

Fruits

Fruits are not only sweet and delicious; there's an abundance of evidence that fruits help reduce the risk of certain diseases. All fruits are loaded with vitamins, especially vitamin C, and a range of phytochemicals.

Enjoy berries, including blackberries, blueberries, strawberries, raspberries, and cranberries. Citrus fruits include oranges, tangerines, lemons, and grapefruit. Melons include cantaloupe, honeydew, and watermelon. Tree and vine fruits include apples, peaches, bananas, figs, and grapes. Tropical fruit include mangoes, papayas, and kiwis.

Fruits are ideal as snacks and desserts and make scrumptious additions to salads. Many fruits can be cooked, such as fried bananas or apples in applesauce.

Herbs and Spices

A little spice goes a long way when turning an ordinary dish into something special. Many herbs and spices contain valuable antioxidants and other healthful properties. They add delicious flavors to food, and many give certain ethnic dishes their unique qualities. The range of herbs and spices available is too vast to detail here, so just a few will be mentioned. Garlic helps to create wonderful Italian dishes. Cilantro adds a distinctive flavor to Mexican food, whereas in Asia ginger is a popular spice. Paprika is the defining ingredient in Hungarian goulash. And, of course, Indian food includes all the spices that make a really good curry.

Oil, Vinegar, and Sweeteners

You may have been told that we need fish in our diets for the healthful oils they contain. In fact, it is not necessary to eat fish. There are plenty of valuable plant-based sources of health-promoting monounsaturated fats and essential fatty acids. Nuts, seeds, avocados, and olives provide good sources of monounsaturated fats. Flaxseeds, walnuts, green leafy vegetables, canola oil, and soy products can provide omega-3 fatty acids. Oils from nuts and other plants are useful for stir frying, baking, and in salad dressings. Choose less-refined oils, such as extra-virgin olive oil or flaxseed oil in recipes where the oil will not be cooked or heated, such as in salad dressings or to drizzle over cooked pasta or vegetables. Refined oils, such as canola, peanut, soybean, or sunflower oils, are best to use when you are cooking food at a higher heat.

Vinegar provides rich flavor without adding salt or calories. Try balsamic vinegar in a marinade for grilled vegetables, cider vinegar in salad dressings, and rice or wine vinegar to add flavor to sauces and dips.

Become acquainted with less-refined sweeteners, such as maple syrup, blackstrap molasses, or brown rice syrup. Consider adding some dark chocolate, dates, or raisins to sweeten your granola, trail mix, and cookies, so you can still enjoy sweet flavors without adding empty calories.

Water

In addition to food, doctors recommend drinking six to eight cups of water every day, as an essential component to your diet. Taking a daily multivitamin will help ensure that you are getting all the vitamins and minerals you need. Be sure to take one that supplies vitamin B12, which is needed if you are not eating any animal products.

Choose a variety of foods from the five main food groups every day. Add herbs, spices, oils, and other natural flavorings, and you'll have everything you need for delicious meals that meet all your nutritional requirements.

Making Changes

Several recommendations have been found to be useful to people who would like to switch to a vegetarian diet. Here are seven rules for a smooth transition:

Rule 1: Whenever you give up eating any dish, be sure to substitute an even better-tasting one in its place. That way you'll always trade up, and your diet will be even more satisfying. Make the switch a taste adventure. Be willing to learn and to experiment with new foods.

Rule 2: Don't be afraid! Some people worry that if they are even one milligram short of magnesium their arms will fall off. Just relax. Not only is a vegetarian diet safe (and delicious), but it is a lot safer than the diet you left behind. There's a reason vegetarians on average live longer and healthier lives.

Rule 3: Keep it simple. Don't count milligrams and don't count servings. Just remember to enjoy several servings from each main food group—fruits, vegetable, grains, nuts, and legumes—every day, and wash them down with plenty of water. Take a good multivitamin/mineral supplement (make sure it includes vitamin B12) every day for nutritional insurance, and enjoy life.

Rule 4: Don't try to do it all at once. Make Tuesday night veggie night. Try a new dish each week, then slowly switch to a vegetarian diet over time. Proceed at your own pace and do the best you can. You get points for progress, not for speed records.

Rule 5: Don't jump to conclusions. During your transition life goes on. If your coworker's kids have a cold and you start to sneeze, please don't blame the veggies. If you're kept up all night by the neighbor's dog barking, and then feel tired next morning, don't blame your new diet.

Rule 6: Read food labels. Remember, the devil is in the details. Exactly what is considered a serving size? What artificial ingredients does a food contain? How about saturated fat, trans fat, and cholesterol? On the positive side, how much fiber is included? Knowledge is power. Know thy food!

Rule 7: Be diplomatic when dealing with others. New vegetarians are sometimes very enthusiastic about their change in diet. But it's a free country—others are entitled to make their own food choices, and you must respect that, just as you want them to respect your right to choose the food you eat. When discussing your food choices with others, it is best to share what you are doing but not pressure others to do the same. Instead, live by example and be ready to help others, if they ask.

Shopping for the Vegetarian Kitchen

Shopping for the vegetarian kitchen is easy and fun. There are four broad categories of stores offering vegetarian options: food co-ops, natural food stores, farmers markets, and mainstream supermarkets.

Food co-ops became involved in the natural food business very early on, so they have lots of experience with vegetarian products. Food co-ops sell their memberships to the public. By purchasing a membership you will become a part owner of the store, with voting rights that give you a say in how the co-op is run. Often they have policies regarding the quality and variety of the food that they carry, which makes them an especially good place to shop. Many also offer educational programs to help you learn more about your food choices. You don't need to be a member to shop there. However, if you do decide to join, you'll soon find that the co-op's discounts are well worth the small joining fee.

Natural food stores also abound—you'll find everything from local mom-and-pop stores to larger supermarket-style stores. The smaller stores typically offer a well-chosen stock, and their employees can spend time offering you advice and making special orders. These stores know their clientele well and will strive to find what you're looking for. The larger natural food stores offer the advantage of a wide variety of items and convenience sections, such as a deli, bakery, or cafeteria. They also usually operate with extended hours and feature many in-store demos, so you can sample some of the latest product lines.

Farmers markets are a growing phenomenon all across America; they usually take form as a once-a-week event. Local farmers often keep their best and freshest produce to sell at these markets. Buying food at a farmers market is a lot of fun, as there is often a festival atmosphere. You'll find produce you might not see in stores and meet face-to-face with the actual people who planted, nurtured, and harvested the fruits and vegetables you'll be enjoying. From the Saturday market in the old Grange hall in little Trout Lake, Washington, to the weekend market on two sides of New York City's Union Square, farmers markets are enjoyable and rewarding.

Look to buy organic food whenever possible. Organic food has the advantage of being grown without pesticides and herbicides. You can often save money by buying organic produce that is in season and grown locally.

Not to be forgotten are the mainstream supermarket chains. Although they do not offer the same degree of variety as co-ops and natural food stores, many are carrying an increasing number of vegetarian options. In many supermarkets, you can find several brands of soymilk and tofu. Ethnic food aisles often carry prepared sauces and a wide selection of beans, rice, and pasta. Don't overlook the frozen produce. Picked at just the right time, these vegetables have well-preserved freshness and are just waiting to be cooked.

Make shopping an adventure in good health. Take a stroll up and down the aisles and you will see how many of the products are familiar to you as you keep an eye out for new items and new flavors of old favorites. When you come upon an unfamiliar item, try to learn something about it. Be willing to learn and to experiment. Most of all, place your health and well-being first by eating natural, health-promoting foods.

Dining Out

Dining out is one of life's true pleasures, with many restaurants specializing in different cuisines and offering unique atmospheres. As more people discover the many benefits of a vegetarian diet, there's a growing trend for conventional restaurants to offer more vegetarian options and for more vegetarian restaurants to open.

Dining at a totally vegetarian restaurant is easy since there is a wide selection of options to choose from. You'll often find that most items on the menu can also be made without dairy or eggs, if requested. Most vegetarian restaurants are accustomed to receiving special requests, and many include dairy and egg alternatives on the menu.

Various ethnic restaurants can be found in many regions around the country. Most Indian, Thai, Chinese, and Vietnamese restaurants have many tasty vegetarian options from which to choose. However, other cuisines should not be overlooked. Often Ethiopian and Middle Eastern restaurants have good vegetarian choices on their menus. Grilled veggie or bean burritos and enchiladas are a good choice at Mexican restaurants; ask them to hold the cheese and request whole beans rather than refried beans to avoid those cooked in lard. Veggie pizzas, pasta primavera, and other pasta dishes can easily be made without meat in Italian restaurants, and they often taste just as good without the cheese.

Vegetarian food is also showing up in some surprising places. Many steak and seafood houses are now offering some rather tasty dishes to attract the vegetarian customer. At the very least, you can get a veggie burger in many conventional and fast food restaurants these days, and you can even order a veggie dog at most baseball stadiums.

On occasion, of course, you'll need to eat at a restaurant with few, if any, vegetarian options. If there's nothing you feel comfortable ordering on the menu, ask whether a special meal can be prepared; specify what you would like, choosing ingredients you can see are already available from the menu. Chefs are often happy to receive such special requests and often come out to relate their delight at having the opportunity to be creative and prepare a vegetarian meal. The result can be a dish that is truly inspired.

Vegetarians have never had so many dining options from which to choose. Look at dining out as an adventure. Enjoy!

Dinner Parties, Airplanes, and Hospitals

There may be times when you are served food and have little or no control over what you are given. If you feel strongly about sticking to your chosen diet, your host will almost certainly appreciate knowing your dietary requirements in advance. At a large formal dinner, you can ask if a vegetarian option is available. At a smaller gathering, you may wish to ask which dishes include meat, so that you can avoid them rather than putting your host to any special trouble. Alternatively, you can offer to bring a vegetarian dish to share. At a barbecue, bring a package of veggie burgers or veggie hot dogs for the grill. At a children's party, bring small veggie dogs on sticks, and dairy- and egg-free cupcakes or cookies, so that your child will be able to enjoy the food. A potluck is a great opportunity to show others how delicious vegetarian food can be, so it's worth making a special effort to bring a particularly appetizing dish or two.

With the rapidly changing market for air travel these days, it's worth calling the airline at least 24 hours ahead of time to ask if food is served on your flight, and to place an order for a vegetarian option when food is provided. If no food is served on your flight, I'd suggest bringing your own, since food choices for sale on airlines are limited.

If you need to stay in the hospital, it is worth letting your doctor or caregiver know your dietary requirements as soon as you check in. The process of providing hospital food is complicated by many patients having special needs, so the doctor may need to authorize your request in advance.

With a little forethought, you'll find that you can incorporate some simple changes into your life quickly and easily, and you'll be loving your new vegetarian diet in no time!

Chapter 3

A Diet for All Ages

By now, you may be thinking that you would like to try a vegetarian diet for yourself, but you may wonder if it's OK for growing kids. As you will see, a vegetarian diet offers children many nutritional and health advantages. In fact, a vegetarian diet will bring your family health benefits at every age.

Pregnancy and Infancy

Healthy moms and babies are something we all want and support. Many women needlessly worry if a vegetarian diet is safe during pregnancy. Study after study has shown that a vegetarian diet during pregnancy is both safe and health promoting. In fact, the American Dietetic Association says, "A vegetarian diet planned in accord with current dietary recommendations can easily meet the nutritional needs of pregnancy."

The main reason why it's vitally important for a mother to cut down on animal products is because of bioaccumulation. Good nutrition for a baby truly started when the mother was a baby herself. This is because various toxic substances acquired in the diet accumulate and concentrate over time within the mother, especially in her fat tissues. When a girl grows up to be a woman, she may transfer to her young children much of the toxic-chemical load she has been exposed to, through the placenta and then later through her breast milk.

Different toxic chemicals affect the body in different ways. Some are carcinogens; this means that they cause cancer, usually several years after exposure. Some are cocarcinogens; this means that they cause cancer when combined with another substance. Other toxic chemicals cause problems in the growth and development of different organs. For instance, methyl mercury causes damage to babies' brains and nervous systems. The problem of mercury has gotten so bad that the Food and Drug Administration has advised pregnant women against consuming certain species of fish, including some kinds of tuna.

Industrial Toxic Chemicals in Our Food (Table 3.1)

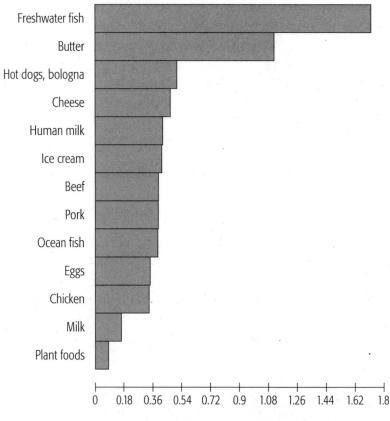

Dioxins, Dibenzofurans and PCBs in our food
(toxic equivalency in parts per trillion)

*Source: Arnold Schecter. 2001. Intake of dioxins and related
compounds from food in the US population. Journal of Toxicology
and Environmental Health, Part A, 63:1-18.*

Broadly speaking, there are two groups of toxic chemicals that we are concerned with when it comes to food. One group includes industrial pollutants such as polychlorinated biphenyls (PCBs), dioxins, and methyl mercury. These toxic chemicals wind up in animal and plant foods predominantly through water and air pollution. Notice in Table 3.1 how the level of these industrial toxic chemicals is much greater in animal products than in a vegetarian diet, which contains no animal products.

Pesticide Residues in the US Diet (Table 3.2)

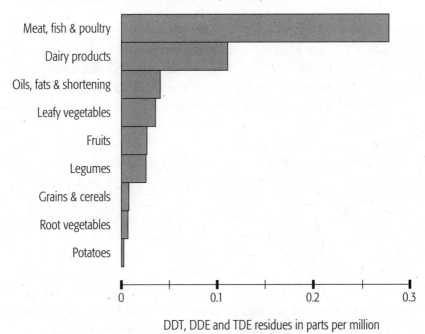

DDT, DDE and TDE residues in parts per million

Source: P.E. Corneliussen. 1969. Pesticide residues in total diet.
Pesticide Monitoring Journal 2:140-152

The same pattern is seen when we look at the second main group of toxic chemicals, pesticides and herbicides, which are applied to plant foods by farmers. In Table 3.2, see how high the levels of pesticide residues are in meat, fish, and poultry compared with plant foods.

Although choosing organic produce is a good first step in avoiding pesticides and herbicides, you can see that reducing the consumption of animal products is a far more effective way of limiting the toxic chemicals you ingest. This not only reduces the most concentrated pesticides and herbicides, it also reduces industrial toxic chemicals which cannot be avoided merely by eating organic produce. In fact, well over 90 percent of all the toxic chemicals we are exposed to do not come from the air we breathe or the water we drink, but instead from the food we eat.

Here's why this is so: when farm animals eat their feed, or fish eat plankton or smaller fish, they store and concentrate the toxic chemicals in their bodies. They in essence become piggy banks for toxic chemicals, storing them all their lives in their muscle and fat tissue. When we eat them, we break into the bank and receive a large load of toxic chemicals. Then, if we follow a diet that regularly includes animal products, we become toxic chemical piggy banks ourselves. When we eat meat, fish, dairy, and eggs, we are consuming a more concentrated source of chemicals, so the levels of toxic chemicals that accumulate in our bodies are even higher than in the animals we eat.

This process is known as bioamplification and is a well-understood biochemical phenomenon. Because of bioamplification, each step in the food chain has a higher level of toxic chemicals than the one below it. For further clarification, see Figure 4.2, page 47.

When a woman becomes pregnant and later breast-feeds her children, she becomes the next step in the food chain and will deliver to her fetus and baby an even larger and more concentrated dose of toxic chemicals, first through the placenta and later through her breast milk. In fact, a woman will generally transfer 20 percent of all the toxic chemicals in her body in only three months of breast-feeding. In some parts of Michigan, women were tested and found to have PCB levels in their breast milk twice that which would be legal in commercial dairy milk.

Because babies take in more food, relative to their size, than adults, toxic chemicals are even more dangerous for them. In fact, some studies show that most lifetime toxic exposure occurs by age five as shown in Table 3.3. If the baby is a girl, these toxic chemicals may later be transferred to her own children. The problem of toxic transfer is therefore multigenerational.

Because toxic chemicals are mostly acquired through animal products, vegetarian women have a definite advantage when it comes to pregnancy and breast-feeding. For instance, studies have shown that long-standing lacto-ovo vegetarian women have only one percent of the toxic chemicals in their breast milk compared to mothers who have followed a diet that included animal products.

Breast-feeding offers many potential physical and psychological benefits for both mother and baby. A vegetarian diet offers a way to maximize these benefits by providing the most healthful breast milk for baby and the lowest possible transfer of toxic chemicals during gestation. A vegetarian diet will therefore not only benefit your health but that of your children and grandchildren as well. Thanks, Grandma!

Average Daily Intake of Dioxin by Age and Sex (Table 3.3)

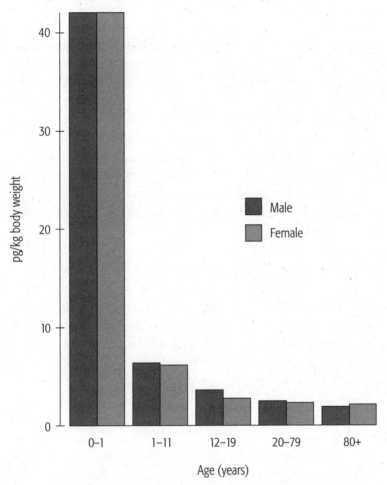

Source: Arnold Schecter. 2001. Intake of dioxins and related compounds from food in the US population. Journal of Toxicology and Environmental Health, Part A, 63:1-18

Healthy Children

Healthy children are the goal of every parent and community. A vegetarian diet offers a child many health advantages.

Type 1 Diabetes: Vegetarian children have a much lower risk of diabetes than children eating the standard American diet. There are two kinds of diabetes. Type 1, or insulin dependent diabetes (formerly called juvenile diabetes), causes the pancreas to stop secreting insulin. Children with this form of diabetes have to give themselves daily injections of insulin in order to survive. This disease also causes damage to the blood vessels. The blood vessels in the eyes are especially susceptible, and diabetes is the leading cause of blindness in the United States. There's a strong correlation between dairy consumption and type 1 diabetes, as can be seen in the Table 4.14, page 74.

Problems Caused by Dairy Products: Most parents think it's natural for kids to drink milk and eat dairy products such as cheese. However, the opposite is nearer the truth. Ask yourself these questions: What other animal consumes milk past the age of weaning? What other animal consumes the milk of another species, such as when humans consume cow's milk?

Many parents, influenced by tradition and the dairy industry's aggressive advertising, believe that without milk their children will not get the calcium they need for strong and healthy bones. You will see as you read through this book that there are many reasons to avoid milk, and that there are plenty of other more nutritious sources of calcium for children. For instance, broccoli, ounce for ounce, has more calcium than milk, and the absorption rate of the calcium is almost double. Collard greens are another excellent source. In fact there are many nondairy sources of calcium in plant foods. See Table 4.18 on page 87 for some examples. Other products fortified with calcium are now widely available, such as soymilk and almond milk. These taste similar to cow's milk, are available in chocolate and other flavors, and are very popular with kids. Substitutes for dairy-based ice cream are also widely available and taste great.

People in many other cultures around the world do not consume dairy foods because they are lactose intolerant. Their bodies are not adapted for milk consumption past the age of weaning. Lactose is the sugar found in milk, and lactose intolerance is caused by a lack of lactase, the enzyme necessary to digest dairy products. Symptoms of lactose intolerance include gas, stomach pain, and diarrhea. Almost 100 percent of blacks and Asians are lactose intolerant. Even among some white ethnic groups, rates of lactose intolerance are over 50 percent.

Rates of osteoporosis are much lower in countries where people consume fewer animal products than in Western countries (see Table 4.16 on page 85). Consider the giant bones of the mighty gorilla and the graceful gazelle, and notice that they consume no milk beyond the age of weaning. These animals get all the calcium they need from plant foods. After all, where do you think the cow got the calcium that goes into her milk? Don't believe the advertising that tries to convince you that dairy products are essential for your children's health. It just isn't true.

Type 2 Diabetes: Another type of diabetes is type 2, or non-insulin dependent diabetes, formerly called adult-onset diabetes (described in more detail on pages 72–76). Why is this being mentioned in relation to children? The reason is that type 2 diabetes is now being seen in children, and the rates are growing very rapidly. Obesity and meat consumption are closely correlated with this disease.

Cancer: Cancer in children is deeply distressing. Children increase their risk for cancer when they consume meat. In one study, researchers found that children who ate three hot dogs a week had 10 times the risk of leukemia compared to children who did not eat hot dogs. Another study found that children who ate hot dogs once a week also doubled their risk of brain tumors, and those who ate them twice a week tripled their risk. In yet another study, kids who ate the most cured meats—ham, bacon, and sausage—had three times the risk of lymphoma. Children who ate chopped meat once a week had twice the incidence of acute lymphocytic leukemia. In that study, eating just two burgers a week tripled the incidence compared to children who ate no chopped meat.

Children's risk of cancer can also be influenced by what their moms ate during pregnancy. A study showed that pregnant women who ate two servings a day of any kind of cured meat had more than double the risk of having children who developed brain cancer.

Cholesterol: Many people think that cholesterol is a worry only for grownups, but meat, dairy, and eggs also raise children's cholesterol levels. The fact is that cholesterol is a life-long concern. Although artery-clogging cholesterol catches up to us when we're older, the whole process begins when we are young. In fact, cholesterol streaks can often be found in even young children who are fed a diet with significant amounts of food containing saturated fat and cholesterol. By their late teens and early twenties, significant coronary artery disease can be found.

Behavior: We all want our kids to do well in school. Many parents are unaware of the connection between what children eat and their behavior and ability to learn while at school. The food children eat has a profound effect on their education. For instance, in one school in Wisconsin, there were rampant behavior problems. The police were called to school almost every day. Many of the students also had trouble concentrating and learning. The school and the children were in trouble. Then the school contracted with a natural food supplier and changed the entire cafeteria menu so that only wholesome food was served. The results astounded even the most hardened skeptic. The police haven't been called to the school for over a year, and test scores have risen. Students with behavior problems also experienced significant improvements, which benefited both the students and their teachers.

Helpful Hints: So what's a kid to eat? It's good that you asked! Here a few hints for helping your children follow a healthy diet:

• It's important to teach children the value of eating health-promoting foods and to set good habits for a lifetime. If you teach them to avoid animal ingredients as much as possible from the beginning, they will get the message.

• Harder for many to do, but just as important, is to set a good example. If you tell children they mustn't eat junk food but they see you eating it yourself, they will recognize the hypocrisy. We all slip up once in a while. Be open and honest about your mistakes and ask for your children's help in improving your diet as well.

• Never bribe children with rewards of unhealthful food. If candy or a visit to McDonalds are seen as special treats, they will only want them more. Favorite toys or stories and visits to playgrounds or movies are much better rewards than food-related treats, if you want your children to have a positive attitude about what they eat.

• To avoid frequent arguments, keep only healthful food in your home. If you are the main shopper, you can control what's in the house. If you resist buying junk food and stock your home with wholesome alternatives, you and your children will find it easier to make good choices when hunger strikes. Fresh fruit, vegetable sticks dipped in hummus, trail mix, and popcorn (not covered in butter or sweeteners) make excellent snacks, so be sure you always have some available. Choose dairy- and egg-free chocolate cookies or cakes as an occasional treat.

• Most restaurants have good and bad food choices available, so set limits before you enter the restaurant to avoid arguments during the meal. Avoid those restaurants where you cannot find anything nutritious that your children will want to eat.

• We all want to ensure our children have fun at birthday parties, but that doesn't have to include loading them up on sugar and fatty foods. Options that work well include grab-and-go foods such as grapes, strawberries, carrot sticks, corn chips, and mini soy dogs. Choose a dairy- and egg-free birthday cake to hold the candles, and serve it with soy ice cream.

• It is inevitable that you will want to share favorite foods from your childhood with your children; just find healthier ways to prepare them. Replace milk with soymilk, white flour with whole wheat pastry flour, and eggs with tofu, mashed bananas, or ground flaxseeds (and use a little extra baking powder to help cakes rise), and you will be able to create delicious versions of Grandma's original recipes. Today's natural food stores offer a great selection of veggie hot dogs, veggie burgers, and even sliced veggie ham, bologna, and turkey for sandwiches. A soy dog with yellow mustard during a ball game tastes delicious.

The Teenage Years

This is a time when many young people first become aware of vegetarianism and develop and interest in becoming a vegetarian. They have many of the same reasons as adults for this decision, but they also have an extra one: rebelling against their parents and what used to be called "the establishment." Many parents worry about their teens when this happens. However, parents can rest assured that becoming a vegetarian is one of the smartest rebellions their kids will ever make, even if the kids themselves are unaware of it.

Cholesterol: It's never too early to start thinking about cholesterol and your arteries. The process that results in clogged coronary arteries, the cause of heart attacks, may catch up with us in our later years, but it begins very early. By following a vegetarian diet, teens will have the opportunity to avoid many major health issues (see pages 50–58). Professor William S. Collins describes one example of this: "American men killed in the Korean War showed, even at the age of 22, striking signs of arteriosclerotic disease in their hearts, as compared with Korean soldiers who were free of this damage to their blood vessels. The Americans were fed plenty of milk, butter, eggs, and meat. The Koreans were basically vegetarians."

Acne: While teens are generally thought of as indestructible, they do still have some health concerns. Acne, while not life-threatening, is often thought of as a fate worse than death by many teens. A very interesting study showed a strong link between dairy consumption and acne in teens.

Healthy bones: Many teenage girls are encouraged to drink dairy for strong bones, but this may not be the best way to go. As mentioned on page 38, quite a number studies point to the fact milk does not provide the support you might think for the growing bones of kids and teens. The mere presence of calcium in milk doesn't automatically translate into bone health, since other substances in milk prevent the calcium from being absorbed effectively. It is also important to remember that virtually all milk and cheese come with a high dose of cholesterol and saturated fat.

Menstruation: A delicate health concern of teenage girls is menstrual cramps and PMS. Medical researchers have found that a low-fat vegetarian diet significantly reduces menstrual cramps and PMS in most girls.

A related concern is the age of menarche, the age at which a girl has her first menstrual period. This age has been steadily declining over the past 100 years or so. A diet that includes increasing amounts of meat, dairy, and eggs may be one of the reasons for this change. Growing up too soon has both behavioral and physiological consequences. The declining age of menarche may have an effect on a girl's future psychological development and physical health. In particular, it may be a factor in the risk of developing breast cancer. Many doctors are quite worried about it.

Asthma: Another problem that often begins in the teen years is asthma. In one study, patients were placed on a vegetarian diet that also excluded dairy and eggs. The results were striking. Seventy-one percent reported improvement in their asthma after only four months. Ninety-two percent reported improvement after one year. And in almost all cases, improvement was so substantial that medication could be withdrawn or drastically reduced.

There is one thing parents will want to watch out for when their teen turns veggie. While a lunch consisting of Diet Coca-Cola and potato chips is technically vegetarian, that's not what's recommended. Teach your kids to remember the five main food groups: fruits, vegetables, grains, legumes, and nuts. Use a daily multivitamin/mineral supplement that contains vitamin B12. Also, look for healthy snacks and party food that are available in natural food stores. Because the teenage years are a time when social acceptance and peer pressure loom large in the lives of young people, nutritious "junk food" will help your teen not only stay healthy, but also feel more comfortable around other kids.

Your teens need your support during this time in their lives, and this is especially important for teens switching to a vegetarian diet. Famous role models can help. Show your teen the list of famous vegetarians listed on page 20. It includes many well-known athletes, from Super Bowl MVPs to Olympic gold medalists. Acclaimed musicians, movie stars, scientists, and statesmen round out the lineup of inspiring vegetarian role models.

Winning the Race on a Vegetarian Diet

Can someone be a winning athlete on a vegetarian diet? The answer is a gold-medal yes! Medical studies have shown that protein from the veggie world is just as valuable for an athlete as protein from meat. This is true, by the way, not just for athletes but for everyday folks and at all ages, too.

While a vegetarian diet has been shown to be just as effective as animal protein in building muscle, it has been shown to be even more effective in building endurance. In one study, athletes were rotated through three different diets, with their endurance tested on each. The results showed that athletes on a healthful vegetarian diet had three times the endurance as athletes on a meat-centered diet. As you can see in Table 3.4, the more closely the athletes followed a vegetarian diet, the greater their endurance.

Vegetarian Athletes Have Greater Endurance (Table 3.4)

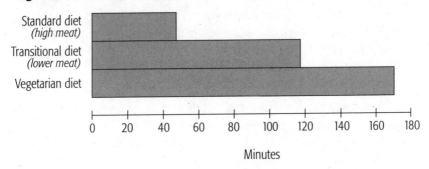

Source: Per Olaf Astrand. 1968. Nutrition Today 3(2):9-11

The names of famous vegetarian athletes abound. Bill Pearl, Mr. Universe and Mr. America, built his muscles on a vegetarian diet. Johnny Weismuller, the original Tarzan of movie fame, won two Olympic gold medals in swimming and credited his vegetarian diet as part of the reason he won. Hank Aaron, who holds the record for the most home runs in a season, did it all on a vegetarian diet, and so did Super Bowl MVP Desmond Howard. For tennis greats Billy Jean King and Martina Navratilova, it was game, set, and match—all on a vegetarian diet. Perhaps the most impressive are Carl Lewis, a strict vegetarian who doesn't even consume dairy or eggs, winner of nine Olympic gold medals in track and field, and Dave Scott, three-time winner of the Hawaii Ironman Triathlon and a vegetarian, who is considered by many to be the fittest man on earth. Athletes and would-be athletes can check out the national organization of vegetarian athletes at www.OrganicAthlete.org to learn more.

In 1999, Scott Jurek, then age 25, became the youngest man ever to win the prestigious Western States 100 Mile Endurance Run. He went on to be the only seven-time consecutive winner. What did he eat to win all those races? Scott Jurek follows a vegetarian diet consisting of fruits, vegetables, grains, nuts, and legumes.

According to Scott Jurek, for an athlete, just as for anyone else, it is important to get a properly balanced diet consisting of whole foods in sufficient quantity in accordance with the amount of exercise you do. Calorie needs vary depending on the mode, amount, and intensity of exercise; even when resting, an athlete's metabolism can be up to 30 percent greater than a nonathlete's. Some athletes can need as much as 4,000 to 8,000 calories per day. A number of vegetarian athletes complain of decreased energy and blame this on a lack of protein. Although it's possible that they are not eating enough high-protein foods, it is much more likely that they simply need more calories. (See Table 1.2 on page 18, for more information.) If they are not getting enough calories, the body may be forced to use protein for fuel, instead of using it to build a stronger and healthier body. Carbohydrates and fats are the best sources of calories for fuel, while protein, minerals, and vitamins are essential for construction, repair, and healthy functioning of the body. To reach their peak performance, athletes will get all of these essential ingredients by eating plenty of fruits, vegetables, grains, nuts, and legumes.

As a vegetarian athlete, you will not only be setting yourself up to win the game of sports, you'll also be stacking the odds in your favor for winning a longer and healthier game of life.

Adults and Seniors

Throughout this book you will see that following a vegetarian diet is unquestionably the most healthful choice you can make. In the next chapter, you'll learn how a vegetarian diet helps prevent and aids in the treatment of many common diseases of concern to adults of all ages.

Chapter 4

Common Diseases

Many people are shocked when they hear how much meat, fish, dairy, and eggs Americans consume every year. The average American eats 271 pounds of meat, 16 pounds of fish, 254 eggs, 180 pounds of milk, 32 pounds of cheese, 25 pounds of ice cream, 10 pounds of cream, and 8 pounds of yogurt every year. No wonder our cholesterol levels have hit the roof! Does anyone think we can eat that much saturated fat and cholesterol and not get sick?

The consumption of animal products has intensified in recent years. In the United States, cheese, cream, and yogurt consumption has more than doubled per person in the past 25 years. Meat consumption has risen 32 percent in the past 40 years, and fish consumption has risen 60 percent during the same time. The consumption of eggs has risen 12 percent in just the last 10 years. Tables 4.1 through 4.4 show the rise in animal product consumption in the United States.

Accompanying the increased consumption of animal-based foods is a rise in many diseases that are considered to be related to diet: heart disease, high blood pressure, stroke, cancer, diabetes, and obesity. In 1995, a study published in the *Journal of Preventative Medicine* determined that the total health care costs attributable to meat consumption were as high as $61.4 billion (in 1992 dollars). Given the high rate of inflation of health care costs, this figure could easily be over $100 billion today.

Other countries have also greatly increased their meat consumption. The worldwide per capita meat consumption has more than doubled during the last 50 years. In some countries, such as China, it has risen even faster. In the 17 years between 1977 and 1994, per capita meat consumption in China actually quadrupled! According to an article in the *British Medical Journal*, the people of China are becoming overweight and obese at an alarming rate, with the country experiencing a 28-fold increase in obesity over a 15-year period from 1985 to 2000. The largest epidemiological study ever conducted, which looked at the connection between diet and disease, was the China Study, led

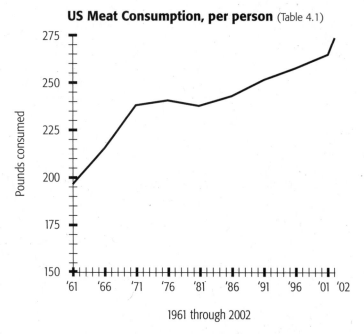

US Meat Consumption, per person (Table 4.1)

1961 through 2002

Source: Food and Agriculture Organization of the United Nations (FAO). 2004. FAOSTAT Online Statistical Service.

by Dr. T. Colin Campbell, Professor Emeritus of Nutritional Biochemistry at Cornell University. This study correlated the rise in a number of common diseases with the rise in consumption of animal products.

A similar trend is occurring in many other countries. This is what Dr. Ethel R. Nelson, a noted pathologist, said about her findings in Thailand, "A study which I conducted on patients treated for heart attacks in Bangkok, Thailand, showed an enormous increase in coronary heart disease during the past 20 years."

Diabetes rates in the developing world are climbing too. For instance, in 2003 over 20 percent of the people in the United Arab Emirates had diabetes. The number of people with diabetes is expected to double in the next 15 years in Africa, and increase by 85 percent in Latin America. The same trends exist for cancer and several other diseases, corresponding with a rise in the consumption of animal-based foods.

In his book *Reversing Heart Disease,* cardiologist Dean Ornish sums up the value of a vegetarian diet as follows: "More evidence is accumulating that a low-fat vegetarian diet may not only help prevent the onset of heart

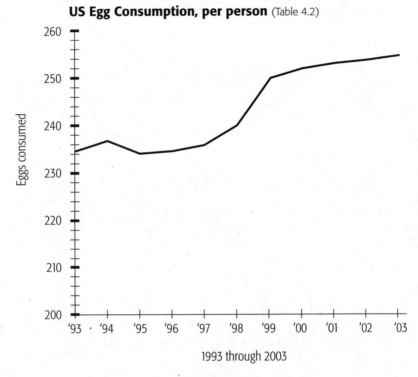

US Egg Consumption, per person (Table 4.2)

1993 through 2003

Source: Egg Industry Fact Sheet. Revised February 2004.

disease and stroke but also some of the most common cancers including breast, prostate, colon, lung, and ovarian cancers. Vegetarians also have lower rates of osteoporosis, adult-onset diabetes, hypertension, obesity, and many other illnesses."

There's a common saying: What's old is new. Hippocrates (460–357 BC), known as the "father of medicine", said "He who does not know food, how can he understand the disease of man?" Doctors both ancient and modern have understood that diet is one of the keys to understanding and preventing disease.

Many prevalent modern diseases (such as heart disease, stroke, some cancers, obesity, and others) have been largely self-inflicted. The good news is that we may also have the power to undo some of this damage by following a vegetarian diet. That simple, affordable, and delicious vegetarian meal may very well turn out to be the twenty-first century's most powerful medicine to both prevent and help cure the diseases of modern life.

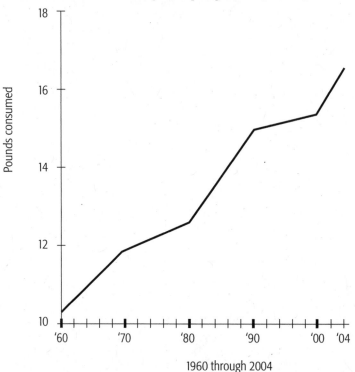

US Fish Consumption, per person (Table 4.3)

Source: National Marine Fisheries Service. US annual per capita consumption of commercial fish and shellfish 1910-2004.

The Shifting Paradigm: The Times They Are a-Changin'

Over the years, many articles in medical journals reported on research done to determine whether or not people could be healthy on a vegetarian diet. This raised concern that a vegetarian diet might be risky in some way. Current medical research has proven these concerns to not only be unfounded but unwarranted. The paradigm has definitely shifted. In fact, it has done a complete about face. Dr. Marion Nestle, chair of the nutrition department at New York University, says, "There's no question that largely vegetarian diets are as healthy as you can get. The evidence is so strong and overwhelming, and produced over such a long period of time, that it's no longer debatable."

The new focus of medical research is on how many diseases can be prevented and how many more years a vegetarian diet can extend our lives.

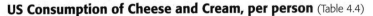

US Consumption of Cheese and Cream, per person (Table 4.4)

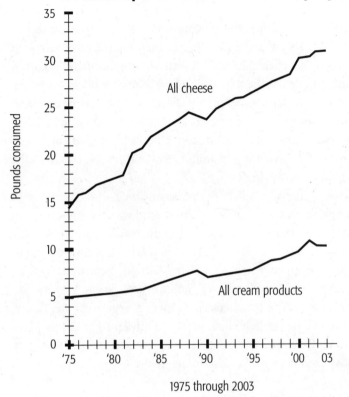

1975 through 2003

Source: USDA Economic Research Service. 2004. Livestock, Dairy and Poultry Outlook. June 29th 2004.

Dr. Joan Sabate, chair of the Department of Nutrition at Loma Linda University School of Public Health, sums it up as follows, "During the past 20 years, scores of nutritional studies have documented the benefits of vegetarian and other plant-based diets, namely a reduction of risk for many chronic degenerative diseases and total mortality. Vegetarians living in affluent countries enjoy remarkably good health, exemplified by low rates of obesity, coronary diseases, diabetes, and many cancers, and increased longevity."

There are two main reasons for the robust health advantages that vegetarians enjoy. First, by eliminating animal-based foods, vegetarians avoid many of the common diseases associated with their consumption. Second, the plant-based foods that make up a vegetarian diet—fruits, vegetables, grains, nuts, and legumes—have properties that provide protection from a wide variety of diseases.

There's a second paradigm shift emerging—the realization that we should put a greater emphasis on prevention rather than treatment of common chronic diseases such as heart disease, hypertension, cancer, and diabetes. Dr. Denis Burkitt, recipient of the gold medal of the British Medical Association, put it very well when he said, "If people are falling over the edge of a cliff and sustaining injuries, the problem could be dealt with by stationing ambulances at the bottom, or erecting a fence at the top. Unfortunately, we put far too much effort into the provisioning of ambulances and far too little into the simple approach of erecting fences."

Dr. J. Wayne McFarland, fellow of the Mayo Clinic, said, "It will be in the field of nutrition that some of our greatest strides in the prevention of disease will yet come. Here preventative medicine reaches its zenith, since food has to do with the very essence of life itself. It is the fuel that maintains, repairs, and runs the human machine. It is the source of the material needed to keep the body tissue healthy, vigorous, and free of sickness."

The evidence is in. The paradigm has shifted. A vegetarian diet is now widely recognized as the key ingredient in preventative medicine. It requires no prescription, costs no extra money, and helps prevent a long list of diseases. The preventative medicine of a vegetarian diet never tasted so good!

Getting to the Heart of the Matter

Your heart is an amazing organ. It continuously pumps oxygen and nutrient-rich blood throughout your body to sustain your life. This fist-sized powerhouse beats (expands and contracts) 100,000 times per day, pumping five or six quarts of blood each minute, or about 2,000 gallons per day. As the heart beats, it pumps blood through a system of vessels, elastic tubes that carry blood to every part of the body, including the heart itself. The flow of blood is essential to our lives. It brings oxygen and nutrients to every organ and tissue of the body, and removes waste products as it circulates.

Although the heart's chambers are full of the blood that is being pumped, the heart itself receives no nourishment from this blood. The heart receives its own supply of blood from a network of arteries called the coronary arteries.

Coronary artery disease affects almost 13 million Americans, making it the most common form of heart disease. It is caused by a condition known as atherosclerosis, which happens when a waxy substance, called plaque, forms inside the coronary arteries. This substance is made of cholesterol, fatty compounds, calcium, and a blood-clotting material called fibrin.

Scientists think atherosclerosis starts when the inner lining of the artery is damaged. High blood pressure, high levels of cholesterol and triglycerides in the blood, and smoking are believed to lead to the development of plaque. When arteries are clogged with plaque, they become narrow, thus restricting blood flow to the heart and other organs. Without adequate blood supply, the heart becomes starved of the oxygen and vital nutrients it needs to work properly. If blood flow is very severely restricted, a heart attack may result.

Coronary artery disease and its complications, such as heart attack, are the leading causes of death in the United States. Annually, more than one

How Arteries Become Clogged (Figure 4.1)

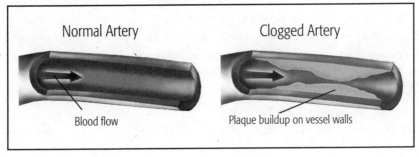

Normal Artery · Blood flow

Clogged Artery · Plaque buildup on vessel walls

million people in the U.S. have a heart attack, and about half of them die from it.

Angina pectoris is the medical term for chest pain or discomfort due to coronary artery disease. Angina occurs when the heart muscle doesn't get as much blood (hence as much oxygen) as it needs. This usually happens because one or more of the coronary arteries is narrowed or blocked by plaque. Approximately 6.8 million Americans are diagnosed with angina every year, about 4.2 million of whom are women.

Once the coronary arteries are clogged, bypass surgery is the usual treatment. This surgery involves removing a section of a blood vessel from another part of the body and sewing it to the diseased coronary artery in order to bypass the damage. This creates a new route for blood to flow so that the heart muscle will get the oxygen-rich blood it needs to work properly. During bypass surgery, the breastbone (sternum) is divided, the heart is stopped, and blood is sent through a heart-lung machine.

But this surgery does not necessarily "cure" the patient. The grafted arteries that are placed during bypass surgery are also prone to clogging. In fact, half of all bypass grafts will clog in only 5 to 10 years if the patient continues following a diet containing saturated fat and cholesterol. Before that point, expensive cholesterol-lowering drugs may be prescribed. These drugs can have serious side effects.

More than 500,000 bypass procedures are performed each year in the United States, making it the most frequently performed major surgery in the country. In addition, pharmacists are dispensing cholesterol-lowering drugs right and left. Isn't there any way to avoid this sad state of suffering, surgery, and side effects? The answer is yes!

Cholesterol is a fat-soluble substance that is converted in the body to a variety of essential hormones, bile acids, and provitamin D. There are two types of cholesterol, HDL (the good type) and LDL (the bad type), although generally people worry about the ratio of the two. Excess cholesterol gets into our blood in two ways: the saturated fat found in meat, poultry, dairy, and eggs promotes the manufacture of cholesterol in the liver, and the cholesterol found naturally in meat, eggs, and dairy foods finds its way directly into the blood.

Cholesterol is not needed in the diet at all, since the liver manufactures all we need. The optimal amount of cholesterol in the diet is zero. However, all animal products, even low-fat versions, contain cholesterol. In practical terms, 100 milligrams of cholesterol are found in four ounces of beef, four ounces of chicken, half an egg, or three cups of milk. Every 100 milligrams of cholesterol in a person's daily diet adds roughly five points to the total cholesterol level in the blood. Many Americans consume 500 to 600 milligrams of cholesterol each day. While some of this cholesterol can be excreted, the remainder is deposited in the tissues, where it remains intact in the body for years, causing blockages and inflammation.

You can see from Table 4.5 that even so-called healthful animal products contain plenty of cholesterol, whereas all plant foods, including oils, contain none.

Now take a look at Table 4.6, which shows the levels of saturated fat in various fats and oils. As you can see, animal products have a much higher

Cholesterol Content of Various Foods (Table 4.5)

Animal Foods (serving size)	Cholesterol Content (mg)	Plant Foods	Cholesterol Content
Egg (1 egg)	274	All Grains	0
Shrimp (3oz)	166	All Vegetables	0
Pork tenderloin, lean (4oz)	106	All Nuts	0
Beef. top round, lean (4oz)	103	All Seeds	0
Chicken breast, skinless (4oz)	97	All Fruits	0
Salmon, Chinook (4oz)	96	All Legumes	0
Turkey breast, skinless (4oz)	79	All Vegetable Oils	0
Swiss cheese (3oz)	70		
Halibut (4oz)	47		
Whole milk (1 cup)	34		
Lowfat milk, 2% fat (1 cup)	18		
Butter (1 tbs)	11		

Source: Pennington JAT, "Bowes and Church's Food Values of Portions Commonly Used" 16th edition J.B Lippincott 1994, USDA National nutrient database

percentage of saturated fat. This directly translates to a higher level of cholesterol in the blood of people who consume these products.

Many people are turning to lower-fat animal products in an attempt to reduce their cholesterol. While this may be a good first step, these products still contain plenty of cholesterol and some saturated fat. The fact that plant foods are very low in saturated fat, and all are cholesterol free, gives vegetarians a distinct advantage when it comes to keeping their arteries clear.

The cholesterol problem is enormous. According to a report published in the *Journal of the American Medical Association,* one-half of all American adults have cholesterol high enough to require treatment. Over 37 million Americans have cholesterol levels over 240, which places them at high risk for coronary heart disease and heart attack.

The American Heart Association recommends a cholesterol-level goal of under 200, although studies show that it needs to be much lower. Ideally, total

Saturated Fat in Various Foods (Table 4.6)

Saturated fat is shown as a percentage of total fat

Animal Fats	Saturated Fat	Plant Oils	Saturated Fat
Butter	68%	Olive oil	13%
Beef fat (tallow)	50%	Corn oil	13%
Pork fat (lard)	33%	Sunflower oil	10%
Chicken fat	30%	Safflower oil	9%
		Canola oil	7%

Source: Pennington JAT, "Bowes and Church's Food Values of Portions Commonly Used" 16th edition J.B Lippincott 1994, USDA National nutrient database

cholesterol levels should be below 150. Dr. William P. Castelli, Director of the Framingham Heart Study, said, "Turning the patient's course of coronary heart disease around begins to happen only when you get the serum cholesterol down into the 170, 160, 150 areas. This occurs only when the diet goes to the vegetarian type of diet." For 35 years running, not a single person in the Framingham Heart Study whose cholesterol level was below this value had a heart attack. Think about that for a moment. The closer you can get to the 150 cholesterol goal, the better your chances for heart health.

Take a look at Table 4.7 and you'll see that lacto-ovo vegetarians (vegetarians who eat eggs and dairy products) and vegans (total vegetarians who eat no eggs or dairy products) have much lower levels of cholesterol in their blood than meat eaters. This is the top reason that vegetarians have lower rates of heart disease.

There's a second reason why vegetarians enjoy greater heart health. It seems that the high levels of phytonutrients, antioxidants, and fiber that vegetarians consume also play a role in their better cholesterol levels. For instance, a study conducted at Stanford University reported that those following a vegetarian diet had twice the drop in both total cholesterol and LDL (bad cholesterol) as did participants who followed the standard American Heart Association diet. The reason was attributed to these extra benefits that plant foods provide.

Cholesterol is thought to become much more harmful once it oxidizes. Vegetarians have been shown to have higher levels of antioxidants in their blood. Therefore, in addition to having lower cholesterol levels to begin with,

Average Cholesterol Levels in Blood Related to Various Diets (Table 4.7)

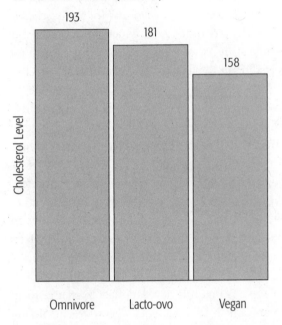

Source: M. Thorogood et al. 1992. Plasma lipids and lipoprotein cholesterol conditions in people with different diets in Britain. British Medical Journal 295:351-353.

the cholesterol that is there causes much less harm than it otherwise might, thanks to the protective actions of these higher levels of antioxidants.

Nuts are another delicious plant food that can benefit our health. Consuming nuts (such as almonds and walnuts) contributes to a substantial risk reduction in heart disease, according to a number of medical studies. For instance, a Harvard study concluded that nut consumption was associated with a reduced risk of both fatal coronary heart disease and nonfatal heart attacks. Researchers at Pennsylvania State University summarized evidence from several medical studies by saying that there is consistent evidence that nuts have a strong cardioprotective effect against coronary heart disease. It seems that nuts are just another delicious way vegetarians reduce their risk of heart disease.

For thousands of years, vegetarians have enjoyed good health. During the past 150 years, doctors have begun accumulating the evidence on why this is so. In 1961, an editorial in the *Journal of the American Medical Association* came right out and stated, "A vegetarian diet will reduce thromboembolic disease [blood clots and strokes] by 90 percent and coronary occlusions [clogged coronary arteries leading to the heart—the cause of heart attacks] by 97 percent."

A study of lacto-ovo vegetarians showed that they have only half the risk of heart disease compared to nonvegetarians. A study of total vegetarians (vegans) showed that their risk of heart disease is 75 percent lower than the general population.

You're never too young to start reducing your cholesterol. For instance, a study of autopsies done on children and teens who were killed in accidents revealed that plaques and streaks were present in the coronary arteries of most of them. Another study showed that 85 percent of adults 21 to 39 years old already have plaque partially clogging their coronary arteries (atherosclerosis).

What surprises many people is that it is never too late to change their diets. Texas cardiologist Dean Ornish took patients who were eligible for bypass surgery and put them on a nutritious, low-fat vegetarian diet instead. A remarkable thing happened. These patients' coronary arteries actually started to open up, even though plaque had been building up in their arteries for many years. Patients began feeling improvements in just a few weeks after starting their new diet. Half of the patients showed improvements in their arteries on PET scans (which are similar to high-tech X-rays) in only three months. Also, their heart's ability to pump blood started improving in only 24 days. As a matter of fact, when Dr. Ornish conducted his studies, patients showed an average of 91 percent decrease in chest pain (angina) and a 55 percent improvement in exercise capability. Some of these patients improved so much they were able to go on long hikes within a year. A few patients who came into the program with such severe angina that they were disabled, were soon hiking in the Grand Tetons, riding bicycles, and playing tennis. Oh how the body can heal itself, if just given the chance!

Dr. Ornish showed the world the power of a vegetarian diet to reverse coronary artery disease, the number one cause of death in America. Other doctors from all over the world have since had their patients follow the same diet and have similarly achieved stellar results. The power of a vegetarian diet to treat and reverse coronary artery disease is now firmly established.

Some people have remarked that a vegetarian diet seems too radical to them. I contend that it is much less radical than cutting open people's chests, stopping their hearts, and putting them on drugs for the rest of their lives. In fact, compared to the usual medical treatment, switching to a vegetarian diet seems rather conservative.

Vegetarian programs like Dean Ornish's are big money savers. A study done by Mutual of Omaha insurance company determined that for every patient who went through a vegetarian dietary program, $5.55 was saved per dollar spent on the current treatment protocol.

How powerful is a vegetarian diet when compared to the standard drug treatments currently offered? To answer this question, several doctors at St. Michael's Hospital in Toronto, Canada, compared a healthy vegetarian diet to a low-fat diet that contained some animal-derived products but included a cholesterol-lowering drug. The results? You guessed it. The vegetarian diet was deemed just as effective in lowering the cholesterol levels of the participants. Because the low-fat diet included some animal products, it needed the addition of a cholesterol-lowering drug to get the same results as a vegetarian diet. In fact, the results showed that the vegetarian diet reduced LDL, or bad cholesterol, by about 30 percent in only four weeks. That reduction correlates to a 60 percent decreased risk of heart disease.

Dr. Frank Hu, associate professor of nutrition and epidemiology at Harvard School of Public Health, sums it up well when he states, "Evidence … indicates that a high consumption of plant-based foods, such as fruit and vegetables, nuts and whole grains, is associated with a significantly lower risk of coronary artery disease and stroke."

You may think that you can rely on exercise to protect you from the risk of heart disease. Exercise is a great thing. Get as much exercise as you can—it helps prevent obesity and its related diseases and helps keep the muscles well toned and the joints flexible. However, it seems that diet, not exercise, is the dominant factor for preventing heart disease. Take a look at Table 4.8, and notice that the average vegetarian has a better cholesterol profile that the average Boston marathoner, one of the most highly trained athletes in the world. That humble bean burrito is more powerful than years of training.

Good "HDL" Cholesterol levels in various people (Table 4.8)

HDL cholesterol is shown as a percentage of total cholesterol

	HDL Cholesterol
Ideal person	Near 33%
Average vegetarian	34%
Average Boston Marathon runner	29%
Average female without heart disease	23%
Average male without heart disease	20%
Average female with heart disease	19%
Average male with heart disease	17%

Source: Castelli WP. "Epidemiology of Coronary Heart Disease"
Am J Med 1984; 76:4-12

It takes time for some people to understand how something as simple as a vegetarian diet can be so powerful. But one look at the long list of medical studies demonstrating the ability of a healthful vegetarian diet to help prevent and treat coronary heart disease might convince you. In light of all this, many doctors are now adopting a "try food first" approach with their patients.

So how does one get to the heart of the matter? The answer is easy. Just follow a health-supporting vegetarian diet made up of fruits, grains, vegetables, legumes, and nuts. The natural goodness of these foods will find their way to your heart to keep it healthy and strong.

Blood Pressure: Roll Up Your Sleeve

We all know the routine. One of the first things that happens when we visit the doctor is a blood pressure check. You can see the look on people's faces as they worry that their blood pressure is too high. Doctors consider blood pressure a vital sign, and they do so for good reason.

Hypertension, or high blood pressure, is one of America's major health problems. Approximately 50 million Americans have hypertension. Hypertension is a major risk factor for several other diseases including heart disease, stroke, and kidney disease.

It has long been documented that vegetarians (both lacto-ovo and especially vegans) have lower blood pressure than the general public. While many lifestyle factors play a role in the development of hypertension, the effect

Differences in Diastolic Blood Pressure Between Vegetarians and Meat Eaters (Table 4.9)

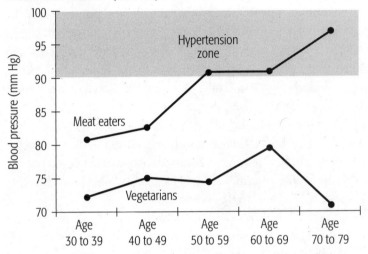

Source: B. Armstrong et al. 1977. Blood pressure in Seventh Day Adventist Vegetarians. American Journal of Epidemiology 105(5):444-449

of diet seems especially strong. Several studies have found that vegetarians have one-third to one-quarter the rate of hypertension compared to other health-conscious groups of people.

Scientific evidence of the connection between a vegetarian diet and blood pressure goes all the way back to 1917. More evidence of this connection was added in the 1920s and 1930s. Studies also show that the blood pressure advantages that vegetarians have are maintained from their teens through their senior years.

For those who already have high blood pressure, switching to a vegetarian diet can achieve substantial results. Several studies show that a change in diet can be just as effective as medication in reducing hypertension. Dr. Neal Barnard, president of the Physicians Committee for Responsible Medicine, says, "Abundant evidence supports the blood pressure lowering effect of a vegetarian diet."

Maybe next time the doctor asks you to roll up your sleeve you can smile and say, "Surprise, surprise! I've switched to a healthy vegetarian diet."

Stroke: All of a Sudden . . .

Another disease closely related to high blood pressure and coronary artery disease is stroke. A stroke occurs when the blood supply to part of the brain is suddenly interrupted due to a blockage (ischemic stroke) or when a blood vessel in the brain bursts due to high blood pressure and bleeds into the spaces surrounding brain cells (hemorrhagic stroke). Brain cells die when they no longer receive oxygen and nutrients from the blood, or when there is sudden bleeding into or around the brain.

The symptoms of a stroke include sudden numbness or weakness, especially on one side of the body; sudden confusion; sudden trouble speaking or understanding speech; sudden trouble seeing out of one or both eyes; sudden difficulty walking; sudden dizziness, loss of balance, or loss of coordination; or sudden severe headache with no known cause.

Stroke is the third leading cause of death in America and the number one cause of adult disability. Some people recover completely from strokes, but more than two-thirds of survivors will have some type of disability and some will die.

Besides cigarette smoking, major risk factors for stroke include high blood pressure, high cholesterol, diabetes, obesity, and heart disease. Vegetarians have lower rates of all these diseases; they therefore also have a lower risk factor for stroke.

The health advantages experienced by vegetarians are not just because of the foods they avoid; the foods they include in their diet help protect them too. Several studies show that diets high in whole grains, fruits, and vegetables help reduce the risk of a stroke. Many medical researchers think that the beneficial effects are due to the unsaturated fats, fiber, plant protein, antioxidants, and phytochemicals found in these foods. It seems that a vegetarian diet is high in key foods that also help to prevent strokes.

A large-scale study of 76,596 women over 14 years and 38,683 men over 8 years was conducted to determine the protective effect of fruits and vegetables. Researchers at the Harvard School of Public Health summarized the results in the *Journal of the American Medical Association* as follows: "These data support a protective relationship between consumption of fruit and vegetables—particularly cruciferous and green leafy vegetables and citrus fruit and juice—and ischemic stroke risk." The effect of nutritious food is powerful. In this study, only five servings a day of these health-supporting foods resulted in a 31 percent reduction in the risk of stroke.

Another Harvard study showed that higher intake of whole grain foods was associated with a significantly lower risk of ischemic stroke among women. In fact, the women in the study who consumed the most whole grains reduced their risk of stroke by 43 percent.

Another study concluded that fruits and vegetables have a significant protective effect on both ischemic and hemorrhagic stroke. One very interesting aspect of this study is that it showed a substantial benefit for even modest increases in the consumption of fruits and vegetables. Small changes can make a big difference. For instance, just an extra three servings a day reduced the risk of stroke by 26 percent.

A study by the Pasteur Institute in France found that each serving of fruit reduces the risk of stroke by 11 percent. For example, based on this study, if you add a banana with breakfast, an apple with lunch, and a fruit cup for dessert after dinner, you could reduce your risk of stroke (and several other diseases) by 33 percent.

Think of every serving like money in the stroke-prevention bank. Deposit daily an amount of fruit, vegetables, and whole grains. Skip the meat, eggs, and dairy and you will have made a sound investment in the bank of good health. You'll be much less likely to find yourself in the hospital saying to your doctor "All of a sudden, it just came over me."

Cancer: Just the Mere Mention of the Word . . .

Cancer starts when the DNA in a cell is damaged by a toxic chemical, radiation, or other factor, causing it to multiply abnormally. Eventually, the growing tumor invades nearby healthy tissues and may also release some of its cells to travel to other parts of the body where new tumors form, a process called metastasis. While early detection and treatment remain vitally important in our battle against cancer, prevention is key.

Cancer is the second leading cause of death in America. More than half a million Americans die of cancer every year. About 9.6 million Americans are currently fighting the battle against cancer. In addition to human illness, the overall costs for cancer in the United States were about $156.7 billion in 2001, according to the National Institutes of Health. Of this, $56.4 billion accounted for direct medical costs, $15.6 billion resulted from lost productivity due to illness, and $84.7 billion came from lost productivity due to premature death.

Causes of Cancer (Table 4.10)

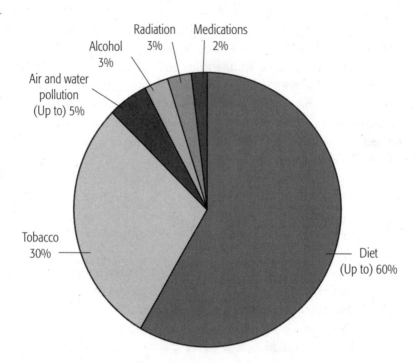

Sources: National Cancer Institute. 1985. Cancer rates and risks. R. Doll and R. Petro. 1981. The causes of cancer: quantitative estimates of avoidable risks of cancer in the US today. Journal of the National Cancer Institute 66:1191-308.

The mere mention of the word "cancer" makes us afraid. We fear what we do not understand and feel helpless against. But the fact is that we now understand much about cancer, and we can do something about it.

Many of causes of cancer shown in Table 4.10 are under our control, the largest of which is diet. Based on this information, it would seem that improving our diets would be the single most important thing we could do to reduce the incidence of cancer. Genetics only account for a very small percentage, and even in that case, lifestyle interventions can modify genetic expression.

The link between diet and cancer is not new. An article in *Scientific American* all the way back in January 1892 observed, "Cancer is most frequent among those branches of the human race where carnivorous habits prevail." More recent studies have repeatedly confirmed this statement.

Let's explore some of the ways in which a total vegetarian (vegan) diet helps protect against several different kinds of cancer. The first way is by the exclusion of meat, eggs, and dairy products. Animal products contribute to the risk of cancer through the toxic environmental chemicals that become greatly concentrated in an animal's flesh and milk. Levels of pesticides and industrial toxic chemicals, such as PCBs and dioxin, are often 100 times higher in animals than they are in greens and grains. Farm animals accumulate, store, and concentrate these high levels of toxic chemicals through the processes of bioaccumulation and bioamplification. (See Figure 4.2)

When we eat meat, dairy, or eggs, we are in essence breaking into a toxic chemical piggy bank, and we receive all the toxic chemicals the animals have been accumulating throughout their lives. The levels of pesticides and other toxic chemicals from the environment have been shown to be much lower in the bodies of vegetarians than in nonvegetarians. Many scientists consider this one of the reasons that vegetarians have lower rates of certain cancers.

Women should note that when they become pregnant (and also when they nurse their babies), they become the next link in the food chain. A large amount of the toxic chemicals stored in their bodies will likely be transferred to their babies, so it's even more important for them to avoid as many sources of toxic chemicals as possible by following a vegetarian diet from a young age. Toxic chemicals in food are especially harmful to infants and children (for more information on this, see pages 33–36).

Studies have also strongly linked the eating of animal fat with several cancers. This may be from the toxic chemicals that tend to concentrate in fat, but it could also be because animal fat, when cooked, undergoes changes that produce carcinogens. One group of carcinogens produced when meat, poultry, and fish are cooked is known as heterocyclic amines (HCA). Two medical researchers at the University of California noted, "There is a general consensus that human exposure to HCA carcinogens is widespread." Even at low doses, HCAs are carcinogenic, and at least 24 studies have now implicated HCAs in breast cancer, colon cancer, lung cancer, and cancer of the larynx, stomach, and prostate gland. Plant fats and oils do not form HCAs when heated.

Another problem comes from meat products that have preservatives, such as the nitrates and nitrites often found in hot dogs. These chemicals react to form nitrosamines after they are eaten. Nitrosamines are highly carcinogenic compounds and have been implicated in several forms of cancer.

The Food Chain (Figure 4.2)

At each link in the chain, the toxic chemicals become more concentrated.

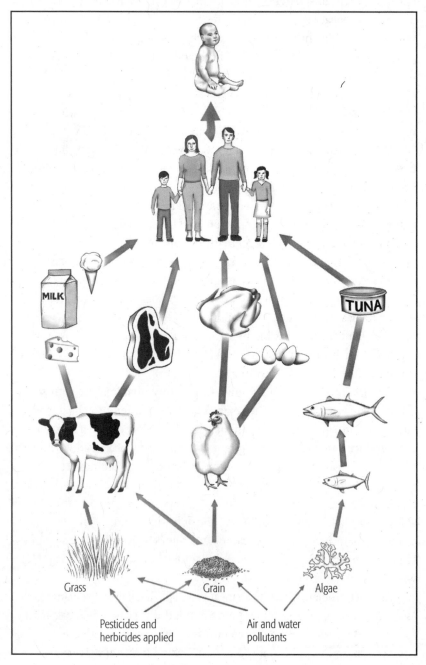

Grass

Grain

Algae

Pesticides and
herbicides applied

Air and water
pollutants

Since a vegetarian diet does not contain meat, it usually contains more fruits, vegetables, grains and legumes. There is much evidence that the phyto-nutrients and antioxidants found in plant foods help prevent cancer from occurring and may even arrest cancer in its early stages. Many studies have shown lower rates of cancer in people consuming the most fruits and vegetables. In the case of legumes, several compounds have been extracted and are currently being tested as treatments for cancer. It often seems that nature is the best medicine.

Another intriguing advantage that vegetarians may have is a better-functioning immune system. The effectiveness of lymphocytes (white blood cells) can be twice as high in vegetarians as in nonvegetarians. According to medical researchers at the German Cancer Research Center, this may be one of the factors contributing to the lower cancer risk of vegetarians.

Let's see how avoiding meat, dairy, and eggs, and having plenty of fruits and vegetables in the diet, contribute to the prevention and healing of specific kinds of cancer.

Breast Cancer: Breast cancer is the most common form of cancer affecting women in the United States today. One in seven American women will get breast cancer. A vegetarian diet can greatly reduce a woman's risk of getting this disease. In a Japanese study, women who ate meat daily had over eight times the rate of breast cancer compared to women who rarely or never ate meat, and researchers in other countries found that for every percent increase in the portion of total calories from saturated animal fats, the average risk of treatment failure for breast cancer rose 23 percent.

A Harvard study, recently published in the *Archives of Internal Medicine*, showed that those women consuming the most red meat had nearly twice the risk of developing premenopausal breast cancer compared to those who ate the least red meat. Dr. Eunyoung Cho, assistant professor of medicine at Harvard Medical School, who led the study, said, "Known cancer-causing compounds in cooked or processed red meat increase mammary tumors in animals and have been suspected of causing breast cancer in humans. In addition, cattle in the United States are treated with hormones to promote growth, which could also influence breast cancer risk." Writing about this study, Dr. Nancy E. Davidson, a breast cancer expert at Johns Hopkins University in Baltimore, said, "This represents something women could take charge of—something you can change to affect your risk."

While animal fat has been implicated in breast cancer, vegetable oils and fats have been proved not to be linked to breast cancer. This is supported by research conducted at Harvard University. In one study of Greek women, the consumption of olive oil decreased the women's risk of breast cancer by 25 percent, even after all other dietary factors were controlled for.

Phytonutrients in fruits and vegetables have also been shown to be valuable in helping to prevent breast cancer. For instance, in one study, sulforaphane, a phytonutrient found in broccoli and cabbage, was been shown to have "mammary cancer suppressive actions." In another study, those women eating the most fruit had a 35 percent decrease in risk of breast cancer.

It seems that total diet composition is important in reducing the risk of breast cancer. Medical researchers in several studies have determined that the more high-fiber foods and foods packed with vitamins and minerals that women consume, the lower their risk of breast cancer.

Prostate Cancer: The cancer that men worry about the most is prostate cancer—and for good reason, as it can have a profound negative effect on sexual performance and urinary function. Prostate cancer is the most common cancer in men, affecting one in six American men. However, leading researchers have proven, once again, that a vegetarian diet can positively influence the course of this disease.

Medical researchers at the UCLA medical school confirm that the data remain compelling that a variety of nutrients may prevent the development and progressing of prostate cancer. Researchers in the urology department of an Ohio university agree, stating, "Evidence suggests that plant-based dietary agents decrease the risk of some types of human cancer, including prostate cancer."

Medical researchers at Roswell Park Cancer Institute in Buffalo, New York, found that people who consume plenty of fruits and vegetables reduce their risk of prostate cancer by about 50 percent. Medical researchers in Taiwan at the College of Public Health concluded that vegetarian food has a protective effect against prostate carcinoma.

Animal fat has also been implicated in prostate cancer. A team of medical researchers from Harvard, summarizing the results of their study, state "Animal fat, especially fat from red meat, is associated with an elevated risk of advanced prostate cancer." Scientists in Japan found an association between milk consumption and prostate cancer risk. Again, no relation has been found between vegetable oils/plant fats and prostate cancer.

Although several studies show that a vegetarian diet helps prevent prostate cancer, new evidence shows that a vegetarian diet can also keep prostate cancer from progressing while it's still in its early stage. In a study conducted by physician and researcher Dean Ornish, none of the prostate cancer patients on a vegetarian diet showed any progression of the disease at all. In fact, their bodies showed eight times the ability to inhibit the prostate cancer than did patients following a meat-centered diet.

Ovarian Cancer: On average, there are 20,000 new cases of ovarian cancer each year in the United States, and 15,000 women will succumb to the disease. Ovarian cancer has also been linked to meat consumption. In one study, women who ate meat seven or more times a week were found to have a 60 percent higher rate of ovarian cancer than those who only ate meat four times a week. In the same study, women who ate ham four or more times a week had nearly double the risk of ovarian cancer compared to those women who ate ham only twice a week. We can see from such studies that even modest increases in meat consumption may lead to large increases in ovarian cancer risk.

Lymphoma (Lymphatic Cancer): Another cancer in which diet plays a significant role is cancer of the lymphatic system. About 67,000 new cases of cancer of the lymphatic system are diagnosed per year in the United States, and 22,000 people will succumb to this disease. In a study of women in Iowa, those eating the most meat had double the risk of lymphoma as those eating the least. In this study, just eating hamburgers four times a week doubled a woman's risk of this disease. In another study, conducted at the Mayo Clinic, those consuming the most vegetables cut their risk of non-Hodgkin's lymphoma by almost half.

Esophageal and Stomach Cancers: Each year 21,500 people get stomach cancer in the United States, and 12,400 people a year die from it. One study showed that the consumption of fruits, vegetables, and whole grains reduced the risk of cancer of the esophagus. Another study showed that those eating the most fiber had as much as a 70 percent decrease in the risk of stomach cancer.

Pancreatic Cancer: In 2006, 34,000 Americans were diagnosed with pancreatic cancer, and there were 32,000 deaths from it. A study conducted by medical researchers at the University of California showed that those consuming plenty of vegetables reduced the risk of pancreatic cancer by half.

Colon Cancer: Cancer of the colon and rectum is the third most common cancer in the United States. Approximately 149,000 Americans are diagnosed with cancer of the colon and rectum per year. A Harvard University study showed that people who ate meat daily had a colon cancer risk of two and one-half times higher than those eating meat less than once a month. In another study, frequent consumption of eggs resulted in a sixfold increase in colon cancer.

Numerous studies have confirmed the beneficial effect of fiber on colon cancer. In one study, those consuming the most fiber had a 50 percent lower risk of colon cancer than the control group. Another study showed that low fiber consumption combined with high animal-fat intake was particularly dangerous, resulting in a fourfold increase in colon cancer.

A study at the University of Hawaii found that nitrosamines were most likely to cause colon cancer in those consuming the least fruits and vegetables. The reason was that the antioxidants naturally present in fruits and vegetables block the carcinogenic action of the nitrosamines. And finally, medical researchers at Cambridge University in England found that those consuming the most fiber in their diets had their risk of colon cancer reduced by 40 percent.

Lung Cancer: Lung cancer is the second most common cancer in the United States, averaging 175,000 new cases per year. The main culprit behind the high rate of lung cancer is, of course, cigarette smoke. Compounding the problem is the fact that the nicotine is so addictive, which makes it hard to quit smoking.

While diet is not the cause of lung cancer, you may be surprised to learn that it can play a significant role in determining how likely a smoker is to get lung cancer. One study showed that eating meat significantly increases a smoker's risk of lung cancer. Another medical study showed the value of phytonutrients in reducing the risk of lung cancer. Medical studies have shown that men who ate plenty of fruits and vegetables had only about half the risk of lung cancer compared to those men with a low intake of these foods.

Swedish medical researchers reported the results of their study in the *International Journal of Cancer*, stating, "The risk [of lung cancer] for those who seldom consumed vegetables was about twice of that among those who consumed vegetables frequently." French researchers, looking at the value of cruciferous vegetables, such broccoli and cabbage, in reducing the risk of lung cancer in smokers, put it this way: "These data provide strong evidence for a substantial protective effect of cruciferous vegetable consumption on lung cancer."

Smoking also causes cancer in other parts of the body. But even in these cases, a health-promoting vegetarian diet is valuable in reducing the risk of cancer. For instance, researchers in Belgium found that increasing fruit consumption cut the risk of bladder cancer by about half in smokers.

The significance of the above medical research can't be overstated. It is common knowledge that cigarette smoking is a very hard addiction to overcome. Former Surgeon General C. Everett Koop has stated, "Cigarettes are more addicting than heroin." It is important for anyone who feels unable to quit smoking to know that there is an increased risk of cancer for those eating meat and a very significant decreased risk for those consuming plenty of fruits and vegetables.

Childhood Cancers: A vegetarian diet has also been shown to be valuable in helping to prevent childhood cancers such as leukemia and brain tumors. For information on the value of a vegetarian diet for preventing cancer in children, see pages 33–36 and page 39.

A Call to Action: The word cancer shouldn't be a call to fear. Instead, it should be a call to action. Most doctors consider cancer much easier to prevent than to cure. A nutritious vegetarian diet is the single most effective way that people can reduce their risk of several cancers. Many doctors consider a nutritious vegetarian diet "chemoprevention" when it comes to cancer. To undergo a round of chemoprevention you only need follow a diet composed of fruits, vegetables, grains, legumes, and nuts.

Obesity: Winning the Battle of the Bulge

The obesity problem in America gets worse and worse each year. The rates of obesity even among infants and young children are rising. A recent study showed that 6 percent of infants and 10 percent of children under six are now overweight, double the rate of only 20 years ago. Among six- to eleven-year-olds and twelve- to nineteen-year-olds, the number who are overweight has risen from 4 percent in the 1960s to almost 20 percent in 2004. About two-thirds of American adults are either overweight or obese. Being overweight is now the norm in our country.

A vegetarian diet will not automatically make you thin as a rail for life. However, it will give you a very substantial edge in winning the battle of the

Adult Overweight and Obesity Levels (Table 4.11)

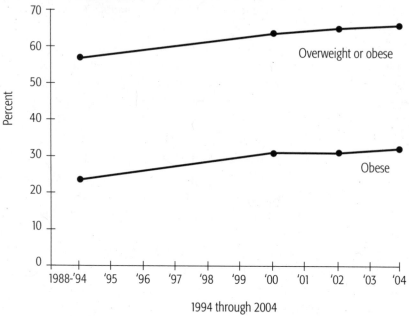

Source: National Health and Nutrition Examination Surveys I, II, and III. 1999-2004. NCHS. CDC.

bulge. That edge is reflected in the lower weights and body mass indexes (BMIs) that vegetarians and vegans usually have.

A study of vegetarians in Taiwan showed that on average they had a lower BMI than did nonvegetarians. An Israeli study published in the *Journal of Clinical Gastroenterology* showed that vegetarians had only one-quarter the risk of obesity compared to nonvegetarians. A research report in the *American Journal of Clinical Nutrition* showed that most vegetarians and vegans had significantly lower BMIs. They concluded that lacto-vegetarian and vegan women have a lower risk of being overweight than do omnivorous women. They advised consuming more plant foods and less animal products to help individuals control their weight. And a research report published in the *British Medical Journal* found that, on average, male vegans were about 13 pounds lighter, and female vegans about 10 pounds lighter, than those who ate meat.

Child Obesity Levels (Table 4.12)

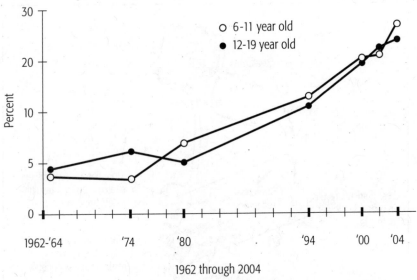

Source: National Health and Nutrition Examination Surveys II (Ages 6-11) and III (Ages 12-17). National Health and Nutrition Examination Surveys I, II, and III. 1999-2004. NCHS. CDC.

There are two main reasons why vegetarians do better in the battle of the bulge. First, high-fiber foods such as fruits, vegetables, and whole grains make up the majority of a well-balanced vegetarian diet. These foods have more bulk, helping to promote a feeling of fullness and satisfaction sooner than foods with little or no fiber. Animal foods contain many more calories per pound than plant foods. This allows vegetarians to eat more food and feel full sooner without gaining weight. (See Figure 4.3.)

However, it's not just food volume that counts; the nutrition contained in the food is just as important. Refined foods, often referred to as "junk food," contain very little in the way of nutrients; hence they are often said to contain "empty calories." Unrefined plant foods are nutrient rich. Our bodies can recognize when we have eaten the nutrients we need, and they send a signal to the brain to indicate that we've had enough.

Table 4.13 shows what the average American eats. Compare this to Table 2.2 on page 25. Is it any wonder that so many people struggle with their weight?

How the Body Tells Us We're Full (Figure 4.3)

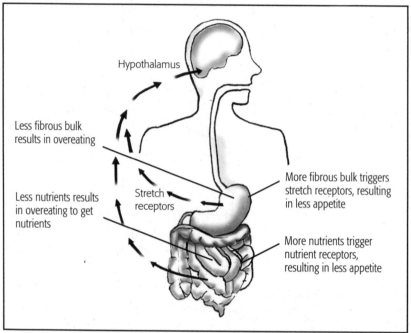

A nutritious vegetarian diet composed of fruits, vegetable, grains, legumes, and nuts supplies plenty of nutrients and more effectively fills the stomach. This combination of factors satisfies your appetite, giving you an edge so you too can win the battle of the bulge.

Diabetes: When Life is too Sweet

Diabetes is a disease in which the body does not produce or properly utilize insulin. Insulin is a hormone that is needed to convert sugar into energy needed for daily life. At one time diabetes was encountered only occasionally; now it is all too common. The diabetes problem is growing by leaps and bounds across all age groups. The statistics are sobering.

According to the American Diabetes Association, 11 percent of men and 9 percent of women over the age of 20 have some form of diabetes. Twenty-one percent of people over the age of 60 now have diabetes. Even more disquieting is the fact that the Centers for Disease Control project that one in three Americans born in the year 2000 will develop diabetes. The total annual economic cost of diabetes in 2002 was a staggering $132 billion.

US Food Consumption by Calories (Table 4.13)

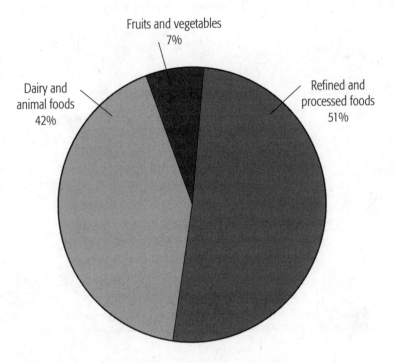

Fruits and vegetables
7%

Dairy and
animal foods
42%

Refined and
processed foods
51%

Source: World Health Organization Food Balance Sheets. Year 1996.

There are two kinds of diabetes. Type 1 diabetes (also known as insulin dependent diabetes or juvenile diabetes) results from the body's failure to produce insulin, the hormone that unlocks the cells of the body and thereby allows glucose to enter and fuel them. It is estimated that about 10 percent of Americans who are diagnosed with diabetes have type 1.

Type 2 diabetes (also known as non-insulin dependent diabetes or adult-onset diabetes) results from insulin resistance, a condition in which the body fails to properly utilize insulin, combined with a relative insulin deficiency. Most Americans who are diagnosed with diabetes have type 2.

Diabetes means more than just taking insulin or medication. The disease's impact on blood vessels damages the body's organs. Diabetes is the leading cause of blindness in the United States; it often leads to kidney and heart disease and can shave 10 to 15 years off a person's life.

Doctors have long suspected cow's milk as the culprit in type 1 diabetes. For some reason, when infants and young children are exposed to

Relationship Between Cow's Milk Consumption in Children 0-14 Years and Average Occurrence of Type 1 Diabetes (Table 4.14)

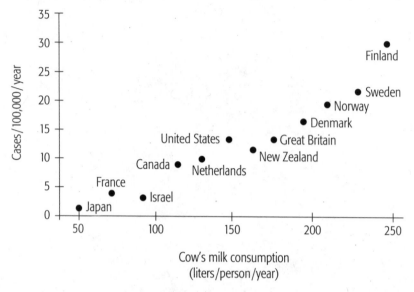

Source: K. Dahl-Jorgensen, G. Joner, K.F. Hanssen. 1991. Relationship between cow's milk consumption and incidence of IDDM in childhood. Diabetes Care 14:1081-1083.

cow's milk, they sometimes develop an immune response that leads to the production of cow's milk protein antibodies. This immunological response can lead to an attack on the insulin-producing cells in the pancreas. Several studies conducted at the University of Helsinki in Finland have documented the connection between the consumption of cow's milk in baby formula and the production of antibodies associated with type 1 diabetes. The presence of these antibodies is a risk factor for this disease.

Notice in Table 4.14 how the rise in dairy consumption from one country to the next is associated with a rise in the prevalence of type 1 diabetes. Moms should note that breast-feeding eliminates this immunological risk for children. Those moms who choose not to breast-feed should know that soy formula is a safer alternative to cow's milk formula for the prevention of type 1 diabetes.

Vegetarians have been found to have much lower rates of type 2 diabetes. Some medical researchers credit the avoidance of meat as one of the reasons for these lower rates. Medical researchers at the University of Minnesota found

Risk of Developing Diabetes as Affected by Eating Meat (Table 4.15)

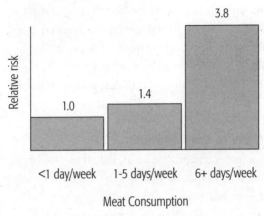

3.8

Relative risk

1.0   1.4

<1 day/week   1-5 days/week   6+ days/week

Meat Consumption

Source: D.A. Snowdon and R.L. Phillips. 1985. Does a vegetarian diet reduce the occurrence of diabetes? American Journal of Public Health 75(5):507-512.

that the vegetarians in their study had only one-quarter the risk of type 2 diabetes as nonvegetarians. They also found that the risk of diabetes rose with the amount of meat consumed during the course of a typical week.

Generally, vegetarians have significantly less insulin resistance than non-vegetarians. As with other diseases, a vegetarian diet offers an advantage due to both the absence of animal foods and the addition of more plant foods. Fruits, vegetables, grains, nuts, and legumes all have properties that protect against diabetes. A study comparing the level of insulin resistance of vegetarians and nonvegetarians, published in the *European Journal of Nutrition,* attributed the low insulin resistance values in lacto-ovo vegetarians to the long-term consumption of protective food. In another study, the diet of vegans in England was found to be actually protective of the specific cells that produce insulin.

In fact, not only can a vegetarian diet help prevent type 2 diabetes, but it may actually help reverse the disease as well. A study conducted at George Washington University found that after less than six months, 43 percent of those placed on a vegan diet were able to stop or reduce doses of insulin or medication. Another study found that in a majority of the patients a total vegetarian (vegan) diet led to the rapid remission of the nerve pain that sometimes results as a complication of diabetes. A low-fat vegetarian diet was shown in one study to improve type 2 diabetes, even without any exercise—that's how powerful it is.

Internist Gregory Scribner says, "A switch to a healthy vegetarian diet can help reverse many of the complications of diabetes, even in advanced cases, and can often prevent the disease from occurring in the first place."

We all want the sweet life. A vegetarian diet can help us enjoy the sweet life with a much lower risk of diabetes. Fruits, vegetables, grains, nuts, and legumes do a body good.

Food Poisoning: Staying Close to the Bathroom

When disease-causing bacteria contaminate meat, fish, dairy, and eggs, the bacteria can multiply and reach large numbers if the food is not kept cold, cooked thoroughly, or kept hot enough once cooked. When you eat such food, illness may be the result. This is known as food poisoning. Some of the bacteria that can cause this disease include *Campylobacter, Salmonella, Shigella, Clostridium, Listeria,* and *E. Coli.*

Every year, one in four Americans will get at least a mild form of food poisoning. Symptoms can include fever, vomiting, and diarrhea. Mild cases can masquerade as a 24-hour stomach flu, but severe cases of food poisoning can prove deadly, especially in the young and elderly.

The U.S. Centers for Disease Control (CDC) reports that foodborne diseases cause approximately 76 million illnesses, 325,000 hospitalizations, and 5,000 deaths in the United States each year. See Figure 4.4, which shows how bacteria most often make their way to our stomachs.

At the beginning of the last century, author Upton Sinclair exposed the extremely unsanitary conditions in the nation's stockyards and slaughterhouses in his book *The Jungle.* One hundred years later, the meat-packing industry still commonly runs highly unsanitary meat-processing plants. Government oversight and inspections are very inadequate. Many people are unaware that only a fraction of one percent of meat actually inspected, even though all meat products may all bear an inspection stamp on the package.

While we are on the subject, you should know that working in a slaughterhouse or meat-packing plant is the most dangerous job in America, resulting in more injuries per worker than any other job.

Unfortunately, the presence of disease-causing bacteria in food derived from animals is all too common. One study of food collected from super-

How Bacteria From Animals Reach Our Stomachs (Figure 4.4)

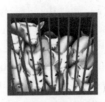

On factory farms, animals are commonly surrounded by their own excrement. Cramped animals spread bacteria to one another

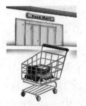

Routinely administered antibiotics create resistant bacteria and become useless over time

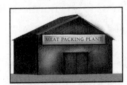

Slaughterhouses and meat packing workers may cause cross contamination

Unsanitary equipment and inadequate worker sanitation spread bacteria to the food for sale

Unsanitary counter tops, cookware, or utensils in the home or restaurant can spread bacteria

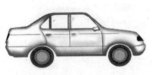

Inadequate refridgeration leads to bacterial growth

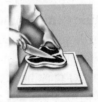

Inadequate cooking fails to kill bacteria

markets found *Salmonella* in 35 percent of chicken, 25 percent of turkey, 16 percent of pork, and 5 percent of beef. According to Lou Ann Jopp of the University of Minnesota, there are an estimated 62,000 cases of infection and 52 deaths in the United States each year due to *E. Coli O157:H7*. In 1993, this strain of bacteria caused the death of four children and the illness of 700 people who ate at some fast food restaurants in the Pacific Northwest.

Also of great concern is that today many of the bacteria that cause food poisoning are super-germs that are highly resistant to antibiotics, making treatment even more difficult (see page 79 for more information about this problem).

Even with new regulations in place, huge outbreaks of food poisoning caused by bacteria are all too common. According to the CDC, there were 22,799 outbreaks of food poisoning in 2003 in the United States from meat, poultry, fish, eggs, and dairy contaminated with various disease-causing bacteria. Even one of these outbreaks can cause illness to an enormous number of people. In 1985, an outbreak of *Salmonella* at a dairy plant made 197,000 people ill and caused 14 deaths.

Usually the only times that plant foods carry disease-causing bacteria is when meat or some other animal product has contaminated them. Fortunately, this is a much rarer occurrence. Vegetarians who consume no animal-derived food products still need to practice good sanitation habits, but they have a substantial advantage in being much less likely to suffer from foodborne illnesses.

This is just another reason to consider enjoying a delicious and safe diet made up of fruits, vegetables, grains, nuts, and legumes. By following a vegetarian diet, you'll be able to avoid those all-too-urgent trips to the bathroom.

Antibiotics: Penicillin Burgers

What do you like on your hamburgers? Ketchup, lettuce, tomato, onion? Who would like penicillin in their burgers? Not too many people! Yet almost all hamburger meat has been dosed with antibiotics.

For many years, the greatest threat to our health was posed by disease-causing microorganisms such as bacteria. With the advent of antibiotic drugs, vaccines, and better sanitation, infectious bacterial diseases such as pneumonia and tuberculosis are no longer the leading cause of death in the United States. But they could become so if the drugs we presently use become no longer effective.

Consider antibiotics for a moment. Antibiotics are drugs that kill a selected species of bacteria, depending on the particular drug used. In any given species of bacteria, there will be some that are quite susceptible to a given antibiotic, others that are only moderately so, and some that are quite resistant. The resistant bacteria may not succumb at all to a given antibiotic.

When antibiotics are overused, most of the susceptible bacteria die off, leaving only the resistant bacteria to survive and multiply. The problem is that the next time the antibiotic is used, it may no longer work, as almost all the bacteria of that species may now be resistant to the drug.

What does this have to do with our food? It may surprise you to learn that most of the antibiotics used in our country are not used for humans. Instead, they are routinely fed to farm animals that are not even sick. Why? They are being used to prevent diseases that could easily spread in the crowded conditions on factory farms. To enable farm animals to survive under such unnatural conditions, farmers must routinely give them antibiotics. In fact, of the 29 million pounds of antibiotics used in the United States each year, nearly 85 percent is used in animal feed.

Humans are affected by many of the same bacteria as animals. We rely on the same or similar drugs to combat bacterial diseases as those used on farm animals. When bacteria become resistant to these drugs, and when we humans come into contact with these bacteria and become infected, we acquire an antibiotic-resistant infection. This can be quite serious and even life-threatening. Outbreaks of antibiotic-resistant bacteria are in the news quite frequently. Many diseases, such as tuberculosis, that were once easily cured with antibiotics are again threatening our health and even our lives due to resistance.

There are often several antibiotics available to treat a given infection. However, since so many different antibiotics are in use, we are now seeing the emergence of multiply drug-resistant bacteria. In many cases, these multiply drug-resistant bacteria are being bred on farms through the routine use of antibiotics. Once they emerge, resistant bacteria can be spread from farm animals to farm workers, and from farm workers to the whole community. In addition, they can reside in or on the animals' bodies and infect people when they consume their meat, milk, or eggs.

Dr. Davidson H. Hamer, assistant professor of medicine at Tufts University, states, "The evidence is strong for a link between antibiotic-supplemented animal feed and increase in human morbidity [disease] and mortality [death] owing to drug-resistant pathogens [bacteria]." Emphasizing the seriousness of the situation, Dr. Hamer further states, "The fact that one's Sunday roast could literally be harboring a deadly and potentially untreatable pathogen no longer leaves any excuse for complacency."

This situation has reached such problematic proportions that the American Medical Association has stated that it is opposed to the use of antibiotics in agriculture, and urges that their nontherapeutic use should be terminated or phased out.

Resistant bacteria are now making their way into our food supply. In one study of food collected from supermarkets, almost all the bacteria found were resistant to at least one antibiotic, and over half the bacteria tested were resistant to three different antibiotics.

The idea of antibiotics no longer being effective scares the heck out of many doctors. They worry that the day may come when their prescriptions no longer work. This is already starting to happen. In one case, a 12-year-old child was infected with *Salmonella* that was resistant to 13 different antibiotics.

In the long run, as more and more people transition toward a vegetarian diet, the problem of multiply drug-resistant bacteria from farm animals will gradually improve. In the meantime, you may want to skip the penicillin burger and try a nice veggie burger instead. In doing so, you'll be protecting your own health and the health of the whole community by helping to prevent the emergence of drug-resistant bacteria.

Dementia: Losing Your Mind for the Sake of a Burger

Of all things I've had and lost, I miss my mind the most!
—Anonymous

Alzheimer's Disease: The most common form of dementia in the United States is Alzheimer's disease, affecting almost 10 percent of all Americans over 65. About 4.5 million Americans have it, and taking care of them costs about $100 billion a year, according to the Alzheimer's Association. The number of people with Alzheimer's disease is rising, with a large increase expected over the next few decades. Alarmed at the situation, Dr. John Morris, neurology professor at Washington University in St. Louis, said he worries that Alzheimer's is going to swamp the health care system.

Alzheimer's disease is characterized by a progressive loss of memory and the ability to think. Eventually, the Alzheimer's patient loses the ability to perform simple daily functions.

Alzheimer's disease is only now starting to be understood. However, it has already been determined that diet plays an important role in both the cause and prevention of the disease. As with many other diseases, a vegetarian diet offers a very significant health advantage when it comes to Alzheimer's.

Several studies have shown that the risk of Alzheimer's disease is greater in people who consume diets high in cholesterol and saturated fats and low in fiber, vegetables, and fruits. One study showed that when past and present meat consumption are factored in, meat eaters face three times the risk of developing Alzheimer's as vegetarians.

Another risk factor is type 2 diabetes. Several large studies have found that people with type 2 diabetes are twice as likely to develop Alzheimer's. We have already discussed the lower rates of diabetes among vegetarians. The same diet that helps prevent diabetes and a host of other diseases in vegetarians also helps prevent Alzheimer's disease. Now that's something to think about!

Cognitive function: Even for those who do not have Alzheimer's, it seems that a nutritious vegetarian diet helps preserve cognitive function later in life. For instance, one study showed that women with the highest consumption of green leafy vegetables and cruciferous vegetables, both high in folate (a B vitamin) and antioxidants, such as carotenoids and vitamin C, usually had less decline in cognitive function than women who ate little of these vegetables.

Another study of 4,000 seniors, conducted at Chicago's Rush University, showed that eating two or more servings of vegetables a day may slow a person's mental decline by about 40 percent compared to a person who consumes few vegetables. The study showed that the advantage was maintained over the six years of the study.

Mad cow disease: Another scary disease that's emerged in recent years and has the potential to affect our minds is popularly called mad cow disease. Mad cow disease is caused by infectious protein particles called prions. The disease is spread when cows are fed little bits of cow meat in their feed that are infected with these prions. The disease invades the brains and other parts of the nervous systems of cows. One sign of infection is a change in behavior, hence the name "mad cow." The danger to humans is that prions are transmissible by eating the meat of an infected animal. When this happens, a similar disease, Creutzfeldt-Jakob disease, or CJD, may result. So far only a couple hundred people have died from this disease, all in countries other than the United States, and new regulations have been put in place to prevent feeding cows to other cows. However, in the past few years, several cows in the U.S. have come down with mad cow disease, prompting questions about how well the regulations are being followed and the safety of the meat supply. Also, CJD may have a long incubation period, perhaps as long as a decade or more, so we don't yet know just how many people will ultimately contract this disease.

If you're already a senior, a health-promoting vegetarian diet will offer you the best chance to enjoy your golden years and avoid diseases such as Alzheimer's and CJD. If you're not yet a senior, you're never too young to start a diet that will help preserve your health later in life. If you follow a diet based on fruits, vegetables, grains, nuts, and legumes, you'll be giving yourself the best chance to still outsmart your grandchildren.

Parkinson's Disease: Steady as She Goes!

Another brain disease strongly linked to diet is Parkinson's disease. About one million Americans are currently afflicted with this disease. Parkinson's disease results from the degeneration of cells in a region of the brain that controls movement. This degeneration creates a shortage of the brain-signaling chemical dopamine, causing the impaired movements (tremors, loss of balance, etc.) that characterize the disease. As these symptoms become more pronounced, patients may have increasing difficulty walking, talking, or completing other simple tasks.

Several studies have shown a significantly reduced incidence of this disease in people who have followed a diet that avoids animal products, especially animal fat. These studies show that people who consumed the most animal fat from meat, dairy, and eggs had three to five times the risk of getting Parkinson's disease compared to those who ate none of these foods. One study that focused exclusively on milk consumption, found that the participants who drank milk faced three to five times the risk of Parkinson's disease compared to those who followed a milk-free diet. However, the participants who consumed fats and oils from plants, such as olive oil and canola oil, showed no increase in risk.

People living in other parts of the world who follow a nearly vegetarian diet have less than one-fifth the U.S. rates of Parkinson's disease. However, when they move here their rates rise to equal other Americans. This has led medical researchers to focus on diet rather than genetics as the main cause of Parkinson's disease.

There may even be hope for arresting Parkinson's disease through proper diet. Dr. M. F. McCarty, a medical researcher at Pantox Laboratories, San Diego, California, has this to say about Parkinson's and diet, "It is not unreasonable to hope that a vegan diet could slow the death rate of the remaining viable neurons, and thus retard the progression of the clinical syndrome." There may also be some evidence to suggest that a vegan diet might make certain medications used to treat Parkinson's disease, such as L-dopa, more effective.

So to help stay on an even keel, remember to follow a diet that is naturally free of animal fats, one made up of fruits, vegetables, nuts, grains, and legumes. That way you'll have the best chance to keep your ship steady as she goes through the voyage of life.

Osteoporosis: Burgers and Colas May Break My Bones . . . but Veggies Will Never Harm Them

Osteoporosis, or porous bone, is a disease that causes low bone mass and structural deterioration of bone tissue, making the bones fragile and susceptible to fractures, especially of the hip, spine, and wrist, although any bone can be affected. There are about 10 million people with osteoporosis in the United States. Almost 34 million more are estimated to have low bone mass, placing them at increased risk for osteoporosis. Eighty percent of those affected by osteoporosis are women, according to the National Osteoporosis Foundation.

According to surgeon Ray Foster, the two main causes of osteoporosis are a diet that is too acidic and a lack of exercise. The acid in most Americans' diets comes from two places: meat, which naturally contains an excess of highly acidic sulfur-containing amino acids, and drinks such as colas that contain phosphoric acid.

When the body receives an influx of acid, it seeks to neutralize it with an alkaline to maintain the pH balance. The antacid that is most readily available is the calcium found in our bones.

A study in the *Journal of Clinical Nutrition* found that meat in the diet creates a more acidic urine, which indicates a negative calcium balance. It is this negative calcium balance that, over many years, results in osteoporosis. Physiological studies showed that doubling the animal protein in the diet increased calcium loss by 50 percent.

The incidence of osteoporosis varies greatly around the world, but many studies suggest that it is related to the consumption of meat. Eskimos have a diet with the greatest amount of meat in it. Not surprisingly, they also have the highest rates of osteoporosis. Studies have also shown that, on average, vegetarians have greater bone densities than nonvegetarians. (See Table 4.16.)

In one study, the average woman's bone density was found to enter the fracture zone when she was in her sixties. (See Table 4.17) Once in the fracture zone, a woman becomes more and more likely to suffer a broken bone due to osteoporosis. In the same study, the average vegetarian woman's bones never entered the fracture zone, not even when she reached her eighties. That's the vegetarian advantage when it comes to osteoporosis.

In addition to avoiding calcium-depleting meats, vegetarians also enjoy the bone-enhancing effect of fruits, vegetables, nuts, and legumes. Dr. Susan New of the University of Surrey, England, states, "A number of population-based studies published in the last decade have demonstrated a beneficial effect of fruit and vegetable intake on axial [spinal and pelvic] and peripheral [arms and legs] bone mass and bone metabolism in men and women across the age ranges."

Legumes (peas, beans, and lentils) and legume products, such as soymilk and tofu, are also important contributors to bone health. A research study conducted at the Vanderbilt University School of Medicine concluded that soy may reduce the risk of bone fracture in post menopausal women.

Because many women believe that milk is a source of calcium, they turn to dairy products in the hopes of preventing osteoporosis. It may come as a surprise that milk and other dairy products are of little value in preventing osteoporosis. A study conducted at the University of Alabama and published in the *American Journal of Clinical Nutrition* concludes, "The body of scientific evidence appears inadequate to support a recommendation for daily intake of dairy foods to promote bone health in the general U.S. population."

Relationship Between Bone Density and Meat Consumption in Women ages 70-79 (Table 4.16)

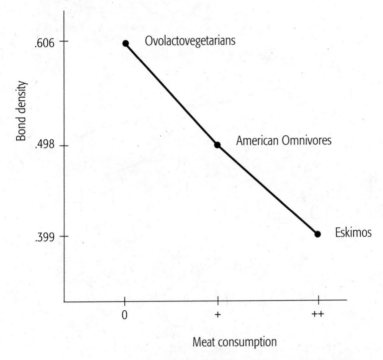

Sources: A.G. Marsh AG et al. 1980. Cortical bone density of adult lacto-ovo-vegetarian and omnivorous women. Journal of the American Dietetic Assoc. 76(2): 148-51.

The value of milk and dairy foods as promoters of bone growth for children is also questionable. Writing in the journal *Pediatrics*, Dr. Neal Barnard states "Available evidence does not support nutrition guidelines focused specifically on increasing milk or other dairy product intake for promoting child and adolescent bone mineralization."

Milk is actually a relatively poor source of calcium. First of all, the absorption rate of milk is lower than many vegetables. One cup of kale or one cup of broccoli provides the same amount of absorbable calcium as one cup of milk. Second, milk contains high levels of protein. As we've already discussed, when there is excess protein in the diet, as is the case for most Americans, the body uses calcium to neutralize the acid. Rather than helping to strengthen the bones, the calcium in milk is used to neutralize the protein in the milk, giving no benefit to the bones at all. It should also be remembered

Bone Density as Women Age (Table 4.17)

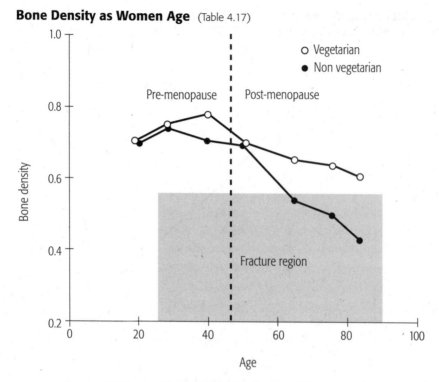

Source: A.G. Marsh et al. 1988. Vegetarian lifestyle and bone mineral density. American Journal of Clinical Nutrition 48:837-41.

that milk and other dairy products (even lower-fat varieties) contain plenty of saturated fat and cholesterol. Milk is correlated with diabetes in children and other diseases in adults.

Some doctors think that the recommended daily allowance (RDA) for calcium is so high because the average American has such an acidic diet. It may well be, therefore, that vegetarians need less calcium than nonvegetarians. Until new recommendations are made, vegetarians should still strive to meet recommended amounts of calcium in their diet, but there are plenty of plant-based sources of calcium to choose from.

If you stop to think about it, you'll see that milk is not necessary to build strong bones. Consider mighty animals such as the gorilla or the elephant. They grow large, strong bones without having any milk after they are weaned.

Calcium Content of Various Foods (Table 4.18)

Calcium is shown per 100 calorie serving

Food	Calcium (mg)	Absorption rate
Bok choy	870	53%
Collard greens	609	Not available
Orange juice (calcium fortified)	320	52%
Tofu, set with calcium	287	31%
Kale	270	49%
Green leaf lettuce	240	Not available
Broccoli	215	61%
Cow's milk (for comparison)	188	32%
Sesame seeds	170	21%
Cabbage	160	65%
White beans	72	22%
Molasses	71	Not available

Source: USDA National Nutrient Database

Arthritis: Bend Me, Stretch Me

Rheumatoid arthritis is an inflammatory and debilitating condition that causes joints to ache, throb, and eventually become deformed. These symptoms can make even the simplest activities, such as opening a jar or taking a walk, difficult to manage. Unlike osteoarthritis, which results from wear and tear on your joints, rheumatoid arthritis is an inflammatory condition.

Approximately 2.1 million people in the United States have rheumatoid arthritis. Rheumatoid arthritis is two to three times more common in women than in men and generally strikes between the ages of 20 and 50. But it can also affect young children and adults older than age 50.

Several studies have shown that a vegetarian diet, and especially a vegan diet, is effective in reducing many of the symptoms of rheumatoid arthritis. Research published in the *American Journal of Clinical Nutrition* and the *Scandinavian Journal of Rheumatology* confirmed that all clinical variables improved within the vegetarian groups in their studies. More importantly, it appears that these improvements are sustained over time, as concluded by a study published in *Clinical Rheumatology,* titled "Vegetarian Diet for Patients with Rheumatoid Arthritis."

Some scientists also have reason to believe that diet may be a risk factor in acquiring rheumatoid arthritis. According to researchers at the Manchester University in England, recent studies suggest that diets high in caffeine, low in antioxidants, and high in red meat may contribute to an increased risk.

Much has yet to be learned about rheumatoid arthritis. However, new information is emerging that suggests that a healthful diet of vegetables, fruit, grains, nuts, and legumes can play a very significant role in helping us bend and stretch in good health.

Gallstones and Kidney Stones: Ouch!

Gallstones and kidney stones are very common and can be extremely painful. Let's take a look at how they form, and how a vegetarian diet can help.

Gallstones: The liver produces bile, a greenish-brown fluid composed of bile salts, fatty compounds, cholesterol, and other chemicals. This fluid is concentrated and stored in your gallbladder until it's needed to help digest fats in foods traveling through the small intestine. If the bile within the gallbladder becomes chemically unbalanced, it can form into hardened particles that eventually grow into stones. Gallstones are those solid deposits that can form in your gallbladder or bile ducts.

Sometimes they cause no problems, but often people with gallstones will have a gallbladder attack that can cause symptoms such as nausea and an intense ache. Treatment usually requires surgery.

Most doctors think that gallstones are related to diet. One doctor noted the following in a recent article in the *American Journal of Clinical Nutrition,* "A diet rich in animal fats and refined sugars and poor in vegetable fats and fibers are significant risk factors for gallstone formation." A Harvard study found that proteins from animal foods may be contributing to the risk of gallstones and that increased consumption of vegetable protein can reduce the risk of cholecystectomy, surgical removal of the gallbladder.

As is the case with so many diseases, those who follow a vegetarian diet have a much lower risk of gallstones. Several studies have found that non-vegetarians are two and a half times more likely to develop gallstones than vegetarians. It is interesting to note that vegetarian foods can also help prevent gallstones from forming. For instance, one study showed that people who eat an ounce of nuts five times a week had a significantly reduced incidence of gallstones.

Kidney Stones: The kidneys filter the blood, thus producing urine. The urine then flows to the bladder and is eventually excreted. Kidney stones form when there is a high level of certain substances in the urine, such as calcium, oxalate, and uric acid. They can also form when there is a lack of citrate in the urine or insufficient water in the kidneys to dissolve waste products. Kidney stones are known to be excruciatingly painful. It's estimated that approximately 3 percent of the adult population in the United States will develop kidney stones at least once in their lifetime.

Many doctors suspect the increased consumption of animal protein as the culprit behind the rising rates of kidney stones. One study concluded that the probability of forming kidney stones was markedly increased by a high animal-protein diet. Another study reported that evidence points to a high intake of meat protein as the dominant factor causing kidney stones in general, and that this factor is aggravated by diets high in dairy and low in fiber. The study concludes by recommending a move toward a vegetarian diet to reduce the risk of stone formation.

The validity of this recommendation has since been confirmed by several studies showing that vegetarians have a lower risk of kidney stones. For instance, a study of British vegetarians showed that their risk of kidney stones in general was only half that of their nonvegetarian counterparts. When it came to studying uric acid stones in particular, another study found that the risk of stone formation dropped by 93 percent in vegetarians.

In addition to the advantage of not containing meat, a vegetarian diet is also richer in those foods shown to help prevent kidney stones from occurring in the first place. One study concludes the consumption of high quantities of fruits, grains, nuts, and vegetables may protect against kidney stone formation. Another study showed that phytate, a substance associated with dietary fiber found in plant foods, significantly reduced the risk of developing kidney stones.

Kidney stones and gallstones are two of the most painful conditions known to medicine, and people who get them often say much more than just "Ouch!" A healthy vegetarian diet, along with drinking plenty of water, is the best prevention for these all-too-painful diseases.

Being Up Front About Our Rear Ends

Around the beginning of the twentieth century, consumption of fiber-rich food started to drop. The reduction of fiber in the diet has had a big impact on our digestive systems and, ultimately, the output of our rear ends. Diseases related to low-fiber intake include constipation, diverticular disease, appendicitis, and hemorrhoids. They have aptly been called twentieth-century diseases by many physicians, as the incidence of these once-uncommon diseases continues to rise to high levels.

These days most Americans only get 5 to 14 grams of fiber daily—far short of the 35 grams recommended. As you might expect, a vegetarian diet is usually much higher in fiber, often supplying as much as 40 grams per day. This translates to vegetarians having much lower rates of these diseases.

Fiber in Animal and Plant Foods *(per cup or serving)* (Table 4.19)

Plant Food	Fiber (grams)	Animal Food	Fiber (grams)
Whole wheat bread (2 slices)	3.8	Beef	0.0
Spaghetti, whole wheat (4oz cooked)	5.1	Pork	0.0
Corn (1 cup cooked)	4.6	Chicken	0.0
Broccoli (4oz)	3.0	Fish	0.0
Peas (3oz cooked)	4.7	Eggs	0.0
Sweet potato (1 medium cooked, baked in skin)	3.3	Milk	0.0
Lentils (½ cup cooked)	7.8	Cheese	0.0
Black beans (3oz cooked)	7.5		
Banana (1 large)	3.5		
Orange, fresh (2⅞" diam)	3.1		
Blueberries (½ cup)	1.8		
Pear (1 large)	7.1		

Source: USDA National Nutrient Database

Constipation: Constipation is the term used to describe the slow movement of unduly firm stools through the large intestine, or colon, leading to the infrequent passing of small, hard stools. Constipation is an all-too-common problem; in 2005 alone, Americans spent over $700 million on laxatives!

Dietary fiber absorbs water, making the stools bulkier and reducing the transit time for food to go from one end to the other. Both factors (fiber and water) act to reduce constipation. Not surprisingly, with their higher intake of fiber, vegetarians are known to be much more regular than nonvegetarians. This was recently confirmed by a medical study conducted at Oxford University in England, which found that being vegetarian, and especially vegan, is strongly associated with a higher frequency of bowel movements than nonvegetarians.

Hemorrhoids: Hemorrhoids occur when cushions around the anus are forced downward. A given stool usually needs to weigh at least seven ounces before it can be evacuated easily and comfortably, yet most people in Western countries have stools that weigh only about three ounces. This leads to a lot of pushing and straining. This exertion, along with the passage of hard, low-fiber stools, is thought to contribute to the development of hemorrhoids.

How Hemorrhoids Occur (Figure 4.5)

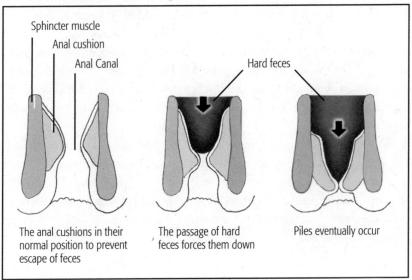

Sphincter muscle
Anal cushion
Anal Canal
Hard feces

The anal cushions in their normal position to prevent escape of feces

The passage of hard feces forces them down

Piles eventually occur

It makes sense that to prevent the occurrence of most hemorrhoids, we need to prevent constipation. According to an article published in *American Family Medicine,* dietary fiber is the mainstay of treatment for constipation and hemorrhoids. Not only can a high-fiber diet help prevent hemorrhoids, it can also help heal them once they occur. A study recently published in the *American Journal of Clinical Gastroenterology* concluded that fiber shows a consistent beneficial effect for symptoms and bleeding in the treatment of hemorrhoids.

Diverticulosis: Diverticula are small sacks and pockets that form in the colon as a result of years on a low-fiber diet. When the colon has to move small, hard stools, the muscles have to contract harder, and over the years pockets form. An article in the *Journal of Clinical Gastroenterology* reaffirms that diverticulosis is attributed to increased colonic pressure while straining at stool in individuals who eat low-fiber diets. Once a relatively uncommon disease, diverticulosis is now very common. In fact, by age 60, two-thirds of all Americans will have developed diverticulosis. When the pockets, or diverticula, become inflamed or infected, a condition known as diverticulitis results. Diverticulitis is a serious disease, and one-quarter of patients with diverticulitis will develop potentially life-threatening complications.

Dr. Walter Willett, chair of the nutrition department at Harvard School of Public Health, found that men who ate the least fiber (13 grams or less a day) were almost twice as likely to get diverticulosis as men who ate the most fiber (at least 32 grams a day). In some studies, vegetarians had only one-third the risk of diverticular disease as nonvegetarians.

Appendicitis: Not as common as diverticular disease but even more dangerous is appendicitis. The appendix is a finger-shaped pouch that projects out from your colon on the lower right side of your abdomen. The small structure has no known purpose, but that doesn't mean it can't cause problems.

Appendicitis is a condition in which the appendix becomes inflamed and filled with pus. Appendicitis is often caused by an obstruction when a hard piece of stool becomes trapped in the orifice of the cavity that runs the length of your appendix. Appendicitis is the most common acute abdominal condition, almost always requiring surgery. Approximately 7 percent of the population will have appendicitis in their lifetime.

Appendicitis (Figure 4.6)

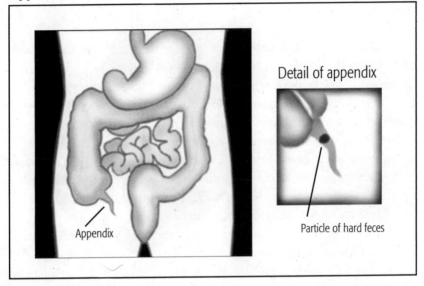

Detail of appendix

Appendix

Particle of hard feces

Again, doctors suspect a low-fiber diet as the culprit. A study conducted at the University of Athens found that those people with appendicitis usually had significantly lower amounts of fiber in their diets compared to the general population. Another study, published in the *Archives of Surgery,* concludes that a lack of fiber may be an important factor in the cause of acute appendicitis.

The best way to prevent these uncomfortable bowel problems is with a nutritious vegetarian diet composed of fruits, vegetables, grains, and legumes, which are naturally high in fiber.

Why Didn't My Doctor Tell Me?

Upon learning about all the health advantages of a vegetarian diet, many people ask, "Why didn't my doctor tell me?" That's a fair question.

Certainly doctors engaged in research have been talking about the many health benefits of a vegetarian diet quite a long while. Dr. Claus Leitzmann, a medical researcher at the University of Giessen in Germany, writes, "A growing body of scientific evidence indicates that wholesome vegetarian diets offer distinct advantages compared to diets containing meat and other foods of animal origin." Indeed, this might be a good time to take a look at the some of the reference's on page 128, where you'll find just a small sampling of the body of scientific evidence.

However, recommendations based on research are not yet being applied by many doctors. Writing in the journal *Atherosclerosis,* Dr. David A. Wood, professor at the Imperial College School of Medicine in London, says, "Progress is slow in the integration of coronary heart disease prevention into daily clinical practice by cardiologists and other physicians working in cardiology, internal medicine, and primary healthcare. This is not due to a lack of professional recommendations on coronary prevention." Writing in the same journal, doctors Christine L. Williams, Marguerite Bollella and Ernst L. Wynder, researchers at the American Health Foundation, confirm that a significant gap remains between physician knowledge and attitudes and the actual practice of preventive cardiology in clinical practice.

For a variety of reasons, doctors have, by and large, not yet incorporated vital medical information about the benefits of a health-promoting vegetarian diet in their daily medical practice. We have seen this kind of delay in medicine before, particularly with regard to recommendations about smoking cigarettes, and it may take a number of years until doctors incorporate new medical information and recommendations into their practice. There seems to be a lag time between the results of research and what doctors actually recommend to their patients.

But you don't have to wait to apply the research yourself. Findings shows that a diet composed of fruits, grains, vegetables, nuts, and legumes will help prevent a wide variety of diseases and will also aid in recovery and healing. You don't need a prescription and a pharmacy to benefit from this research, just a trip to your local natural food market!

What Am I to Believe?

Every day, it seems that a nutritional study comes out to counter common sense. One day it's that eggs don't increase cholesterol, and the next it's that fiber doesn't help prevent colon cancer. So, it's natural that the public and even some medical doctors get confused.

What's going on? Well, the first thing you should know is that the media scours the medical journals for results that are the opposite of what's expected. The old saying is that "dog bites man" is not news, but "man bites dog" is.

That's what most of these reports are. They are "man bites dog" stories. Consider cigarette smoking. Every once in a while we'll hear a story

Man Bites Dog! (Figure 4.7)

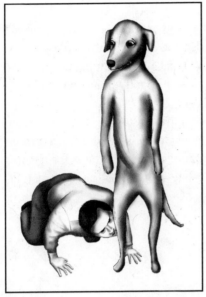

about some fellow who made it to the age of 90 smoking two packs a day. That's a "man bites dog" story. However, a trip to the cancer ward of your local hospital will tell a very different and much more common story.

It's like that with stories about nutrition. Every once in a while you'll hear about some guy who ate fast food bacon cheeseburgers every day of his life and lived to be 90 years old. The media loves this kind of story because it grabs your attention, and that's what sells newspapers. However, a trip to the cardiac floor of your local hospital reveals a very different scenario. There you will find awaiting coronary bypass surgery patient after patient who ate a diet rich in saturated fat and cholesterol. A heart attack caused by arteries clogged with cholesterol is the most common way Americans die; it's also highly preventable.

Sometimes a medical study has too few people in it to reveal a meaningful pattern. Let's say you ask both your next door neighbors who they plan to vote for in the town's mayoral race, and both neighbors say they are voting for Mr. Smith. Would you then conclude that Smith was a shoe-in for mayor after just asking only two people? When you hear about a medical study, be sure to check how many people were involved before jumping to a conclusion.

Every so often, there are studies that are rigged in some clever way. For instance, one could rig an egg study by including eggs in the diet but at the same time removing meat, fish, poultry, and dairy, thereby reducing other sources of cholesterol. The headline could then read "Eggs don't raise cholesterol!" Here is another one. Let's compare two diets, one with 40 percent of the calories from fat and the other with 35 percent of the calories from fat. Thirty-five percent of calories from fat is still too high to get the desired-

health results, but the newspapers will often leave out that little detail. The headline now reads, "No advantage to low-fat diets!"

Always bear in mind that "man bites dog" stories are the ones that sell newspapers. Unfortunately, they are also the stories that needlessly confuse the public. The thing to remember is that although it might sometime happen that a man does bite a dog, it is significantly more common for a dog to bite a man.

Next time you hear a "man bites dog" nutrition story, try to read between the lines and not get too confused. The evidence is in, and it has proven time and again that a nutritious vegetarian diet greatly reduces the chances of contracting many diseases. The "man-bites-dog stories" are better left for the talk shows.

Chapter 5

Global Hunger: The Wages of Farm Inefficiency

Meat, poultry, dairy, and eggs represent the end process of a great inefficiency in food production. When we eat farm animals and animal products, we are, in effect, eating the grains, grasses, and legumes that the animals ate. Since the animals need the energy, protein, and other nutrients contained in their feed for their own energy, body maintenance, and repair, and since much of their bodies are inedible, very little is left for human consumption. Farm animals are, in reality, food factories in reverse. In this fact lies the understanding of a great inefficiency.

According to the USDA Agricultural Economics Research Service, it takes about 17.5 pounds of grain to yield one pound of beef. Figure 5.1 shows how feeding protein and calories to a cow is wasted. The results are similar for other farm animals. For example, when we feed protein to a pig, we only obtain 12 percent of that protein back as pork. When we feed grain

How We Waste Protein and Calories (Figure 5.1)

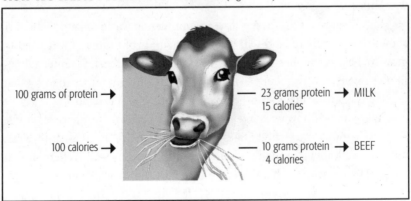

100 grams of protein →

100 calories →

— 23 grams protein → MILK
15 calories

— 10 grams protein → BEEF
4 calories

Usable Protein per Acre 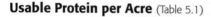 (Table 5.1)

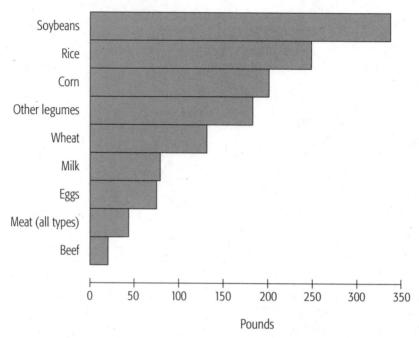

Pounds

Source World Health Organization (WHO)/Food and The Food and Agriculture Organization of the United Nations (FAO). 2002. Diet, nutrition and the prevention of chronic diseases. Draft report of the joint WHO/ FAO expert consultation.

to a chicken, we only get 7 percent of those calories back in eggs. Using animals for food wastes up to 90 percent of the protein they're fed, and up to 96 percent of the calories! Considering these figures, what could be more wasteful?

Raising animals for food is also a monumental waste of land. Table 5.1 shows that an acre of land will yield 356 pounds of protein if it is used to grow soybeans, but only 20 pounds if it is used to raise beef. Seventeen times more protein can be obtained by eating plants directly rather than by first feeding them to animals and then eating plants "second hand."

Take stock of how we make use of the crops grown on American farms. In many parts of the United States there are cornfields as far as the eye can see, and we know that many other crops are grown as well. Where does it all go? The sad truth is that we feed most of it to animals! About 70 percent of the corn grown in the United States is fed directly to farm animals. Eighty

Gallons of Water Required to Produce One Pound of Food
(Table 5.2)

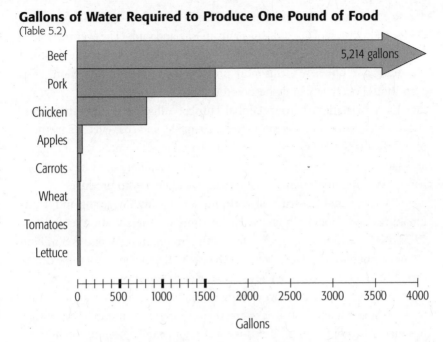

Source: Herb Schulbach et al. 1978. Soil and Water No. 38, [02.10.01.05]

percent of the soybeans grown in the U.S. is also fed to farm animals. In fact, of all of the vegetation crops produced by American farmers, 70 percent is fed to livestock and only 5 percent goes directly to human beings. The other 25 percent is either exported, put aside for seed, or is wasted during the harvest. Worldwide, about 40 percent of all grain is used for farm animal feed.

Raising farm animals is not just inefficient when it comes to food; it is also very wasteful when it comes to water as well. Take a look at Table 5.2.

The availability of fresh water for irrigation of crops is severely limited in many regions of the world. Because it takes many more crops to feed animals than it does to feed plants to humans directly, this is yet another reason why the people of the world must reduce their consumption of animal products. With 22 billion farm animals in the world today, of which 4.3 billion are four-footed livestock and 17.8 billion are poultry (more than triple the population of all humans on earth), the inefficiency of raising animals for human consumption translates to a huge waste of food and resources on a global scale.

Recognizing the glaring inefficiencies of using animals for food, Dr. John Phillipson of Oxford University in England said, "The ever-increasing population requires the rational exploitation of the world's limited natural resources, and nowhere is this more pressing than in food production. Thus man should become mainly herbivorous."

The international group Global Hunger Alliance agrees. They state, "Plant-based foods offer the most safe, sustainable, and cost-effective methods of ending hunger and malnutrition. Plant-based foods do not carry the health and safety risks associated with meat and other animal-based foods. Plant-based foods require much less land, water, and energy to produce."

The scope and the scale of world hunger is truly staggering and heart-breaking. The Global Hunger Alliance sums up the situation as follows, "Worldwide, 840 million people live with chronic hunger, and 8.8 million people die of hunger-related causes each year. Only 10 percent of these deaths can be attributed to emergencies such as war or catastrophic weather."

The global situation is worsening as more and more developing countries—China in particular—have greatly increased the amount of meat they produce. Already the impact of this meat boom can be seen in the number of countries that have become newly dependent upon imported grain. In Egypt, 36 percent of the total grain produced goes to farm animals. Even in Thailand, where meat intake remains relatively low, the share of grain fed to livestock surged from less than 1 percent in 1960 to 30 percent in 1997. In Mexico, the proportion of grain that goes to farm animals has jumped from 5 percent to 45 percent over the last 25 years.

Ethiopia, Nigeria, Iran, Pakistan, and Indonesia are among a host of other nations that have become net importers of grain, fueled mostly by the growth of their livestock sectors. By the year 2030, Bangladesh and Ethiopia are expected to increase their grain imports by a factor of nine, Indonesia and Iran by a factor of four. China will need to import 300 million tons of grain by the year 2020 if it continues to turn toward a meat-based diet. Once the leading producer of soybeans in the world, China is now the leading importer, mostly from the U.S. Globally, 90 percent of the soybean harvest and 40 percent of the grain is now used for animal feed.

As more and more countries start to import food, much of which will go to feed farm animals, there will be substantial pressure on world grain prices. This pressure is predicted to lead to increasing prices, which will hurt poorer

countries and the world's hungry di   As Mahatma Gandhi
said, "The cattle of the rich steal the   ."

  Meat cannot possibly feed the   tions cannot provide
even the basic grains to sustain the   , how can they utilize
land to grow feed grains for anima   aste most of the food
value of the original grain? It makes   at the poor are hungry
because they cannot even grow or afford to buy enough low-priced grain
for sustenance, it is far fetched to suppose that they will suddenly be able to
afford relatively high-priced pork and chicken.

  Of course, world hunger is a complex problem with many dimensions,
including the population explosion, inequitable food distribution, war, and
poverty. There are even cases in the developing world where food has been
exported during famine. These problems need to be addressed as part of the
total solution to world hunger.

  However, for far too long, many in the movement to end world hunger
have not given sufficient recognition to the basic facts of agricultural life.
These facts are compelling and point to the enormous inefficiency of raising
animals for food. It is a fact that for every meat-based meal served, 12 nutritious vegetarian meals could be served. This means that vegetarian food
could potentially nourish many more of the world's hungry. To address the
agricultural dimension of the problem, the Global Hunger Alliance recommends a two-pronged approach to ending world hunger, which they describe
as follows, "People in affluent nations must reduce their consumption of
animal-based foods, so that more people can be sustained by the grains,
corn, and soy that are currently fed to livestock. At the same time, more
resources must be devoted to the sustainable production of traditional food
crops in low-income food-deficit nations.... The solution is to return to the
sustainable cultivation of traditional food plants for local and regional consumption. This cannot occur if land and resources are devoted to intensive
animal-agriculture operations."

  Sir Crispin Tickell, British Ambassador to the United Nations, speaking
at the annual meeting of the British Association for the Advancement of
Science in August 1991, said, "If we were all vegetarians and shared our food
equally, the world could support six billion.... But if one-third of our calories
came from animal products, as in North America today, then it would only
be able to sustain 2.5 billion [in the long term]." The world's population has
already reached 6.5 billion and continues to climb. Worldwide, most of the

quality farmland is being used either for agriculture or to provide housing for the skyrocketing population. Professor Thomas Homer-Dixon of the University of Toronto states, "Nearly all the best farmland is already being used. Most of what's left is either less fertile, not sufficiently rain fed or easily irrigated, infested with pests, or harder to clear, plant, and plow." Therefore, it is imperative that better use of existing farmland be implemented. Using farms to feed people rather than animals is by far the most efficient use of existing farmland.

The ocean is no solution to the world hunger problem. The world's fisheries are producing at a level that is no longer sustainable. Most of the world's stocks of marine fish and primary fishing grounds are in decline. Eleven of the world's 15 most important fishing areas are in decline, and 60 percent of the major fish species are over-exploited. Nearly one of three fish caught are thrown back to sea, dead or dying, each year because of wasteful fishing practices. One of every three fish caught goes to feed animals, not human beings. Only about one of every three fish harvested from the world's oceans actually go to feed people.

Aquaculture, or fish farming, is also a very inefficient use of resources. For instance, from 1985 to 1995, the world's shrimp farmers used 36 million tons of wild fish as feed to produce just over 7 million tons of farmed shrimp.

Another factor to consider is that the world's deserts are growing, thereby reducing available farmland. Raising animals for food is one factor contributing to this problem. The Global Hunger Alliance warns, "Concentrated livestock grazing leads to accelerated soil erosion, loss of topsoil, soil compaction, decreased percolation of rain into soil, depleted water tables, and, ultimately, desertification. The introduction of such operations into nations already facing desertification would lead to hazardously arid conditions. Because drought is an aspect of famine, any increase in concentrated livestock grazing in arid nations can be expected to worsen the problem of hunger in those nations."

The message is clear. If we all reduce our consumption of animal products and encourage poorer countries not to adopt our meat-based habits, then much will have been done to alleviate the problem of world hunger. The food-deficient countries of the world would regain the ability to feed themselves if they could only tap into the largest food reserve in the world: the food we currently feed to animals. The famous economist Adam Smith agreed: "It may indeed be doubted whether butchers' meat is anywhere necessary for life. Grain and other vegetables... afford the most plentiful, the most wholesome, the most nourishing, and the most invigorating diet. Decency nowhere requires that any man should eat butchers' meat."

Americans have a long history of being very charitable and generous. In every generation we have risen to meet the challenge of helping those in need. One of the challenges of the twenty-first century will be world hunger. Every meat meal that is replaced with a vegetarian one means more potential food for the world's hungry.

More than just healthful and delicious, a vegetarian diet of fruits, vegetables, grains, nuts, and legumes is also an act of charity for those who need it the most. Professor David Pimentel of Cornell University says, "If America alone took the food currently fed to farm animals in the United States, we would have enough to feed an extra 800 million people, the entirety of the world's hungry, and we could do it without plowing even one extra acre of farm land."

As is often the case, those who give may also receive in the process. By adopting a vegetarian diet, we would not only potentially make more food available for the world's hungry, but as a nation we would also be taking the single most important step toward improving our own health as well as the health of the planet. The wages of farm inefficiency caused by raising animals for food contributes to world hunger, but with a vegetarian diet there is food enough for all.

Chapter 6

The Environmental Crisis:
Walking Softly on the Earth

There are profound environmental consequences to a world that contains 22 billion farm animals, which is more than three times the human population. Farm animals require an enormous amount of feed, fresh water, medicine, and fossil fuel. They produce greenhouse gases, emit water pollutants from their wastes, and require ever-more living space, resulting in ecological destruction.

Put a Veggie Burger in Your Tank

Consider fossil fuels. Many people are surprised to learn that walking actually uses more gasoline than driving! That's right, walking actually uses more fossil fuel than driving. That is, unless you happen to be a vegetarian.

The reason behind this startling fact is that the average American diet is so meat laden, and meat is so wasteful of fossil fuel. Professor David Pimentel explains, "It is actually quite astounding how much energy is wasted by the standard American-style diet. Even driving many gas-guzzling luxury cars can conserve energy over walking—that is, when the calories you burn walking come from the standard American diet! This is because the energy needed to produce the food you would burn in walking a given distance is greater than the energy needed to fuel your car to travel the same distance, assuming that the car gets 24 miles per gallon."

Agriculture uses 17 percent of all the fossil fuel in the United States, with meat production responsible for the majority of that portion. Since fossil fuel is not a renewable resource, good environmental practice would suggest cutting its use to a minimum. Just as some people make their transportation choices with fossil fuel conservation in mind, many people are also making their food choices with fossil fuel conservation as a priority.

Oil Required to Produce One Unit of Protein (Table 6.1)

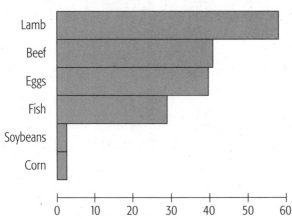

Source: D. Pimentel, L. Reijnders and S. Soret. 2003. American
Journal of Clinical Nutrition 78(3):660S-668S.

Consider how all that fossil fuel is used in farm animal agriculture. Large quantities of fossil fuel are used in the production of fertilizers and the fueling of irrigation pumps. Fossil fuels are also used in the production of pesticides and herbicides. And of course fossil fuels are used to run the farm machinery needed to apply the fertilizers and pesticides and to plant and harvest the crops. Now consider that once the crops are harvested, two-thirds of them are transported with vehicles powered by fossil fuels so they can be fed to farm animals. The animals are eventually trucked to slaughterhouses, and then their flesh is stored in refrigerators and freezers, often for an extended time. All this takes even more fossil fuel.

The fact is that getting protein from animals is very costly and inefficient. Look at Table 6.1 to see how much oil it takes to produce a unit of protein of animal food.

The same thing is true of calories. Getting calories from animal-derived foods is very inefficient compared to plant foods. Take a look at Table 6.2. If you compare the data for corn and beef, for instance, corn gives 60 times more food energy than beef per calorie of fossil fuel used in production.

You can see from Tables 6.1 and 6.2 that the difference in fuel efficiency between producing vegetarian food and animal-derived products is quite

How We Waste Oil Getting Our Food Energy from Animals....

(Table 6.2)

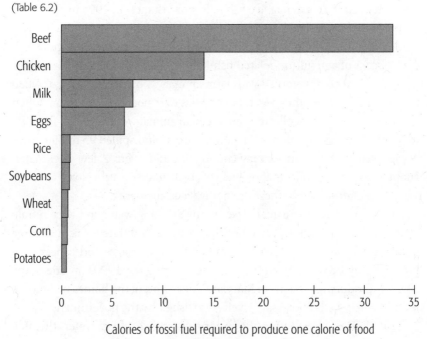

Calories of fossil fuel required to produce one calorie of food

Source: D. Pimentel. 1979. Food Calories produced per calorie input from fossil fuel. Food, Energy and Society p.56-59 John Wiley and Sons.

large. This difference in efficiency translates to the substantial reduction in the amount of fossil fuel used in a vegetarian diet.

Something Smells

How can it be put politely? A big part of the environmental problem caused by raising animals can be summed up in two words: feces and urine. All of that food and water fed to farm animals is excreted sooner or later, and it isn't a pretty sight.

There are 9 billion farm animals in the United States, and 22 billion worldwide, which creates a rather large pile of poop. In total, 130 times more animal waste than human waste is produced each year. In 1997, poultry, swine, beef, and dairy facilities produced a total of 291 billion pounds of waste.

Some of this waste can be used as fertilizer, but a lot is just stockpiled. Look out when it rains! Much of that poop winds up in our rivers and streams untreated and is one of the largest sources of water pollution in the United States. It often results in massive fish kills. For instance, in 1995 in Nebraska, 50 percent of all agriculture-related fish kills investigated were due to livestock waste. In 1996, that percentage rose to 75 percent. In 1997 and 1998, 100 percent of agriculture-related fish kills were traced to livestock waste.

Anyone who has worked with farm animals knows that they "go" when they want and where they want. No one has ever potty trained them. Often the urine and feces are collected and stored in animal waste lagoons. In 1995, in North Carolina, one of these lagoons gave way and spilled 95 million liters of pig waste into the surrounding countryside and rivers. A few weeks later, another lagoon spilled 34 million liters of chicken waste into a North Carolina waterway. Unfortunately, these are not isolated incidents.

Farm animal waste can also get in our drinking water and raise nitrate levels, creating a serious public health threat. High nitrate levels near large farm animal operations have been linked to miscarriages and cancer. The problem may be widespread. For instance, during the 1990s, in one of the chicken-producing sections of Maryland, one-third of the homes had nitrate levels in their wells above safe levels established by the government.

In addition to polluting the waterways and drinking water, there's a problem with all that poop that should not be overlooked: the smell! In addition to the noxious odors of animal feces, the urine from farm animals creates an ammonia-like smell. Clearly there are quality of life issues for anyone within smelling range.

Aquaculture, or fish farming, also generates a lot of waste. Daniel Pauly, professor of fisheries at the University of British Columbia in Vancouver, has this to say about aquaculture, "They're like floating pig farms.... They consume a tremendous amount of highly concentrated protein pellets, and they make a terrific mess." Fish wastes and uneaten feed smother the sea floor beneath these farms, generating bacteria that consume oxygen vital to shellfish and other bottom-dwelling sea creatures. Disease and parasites, which would normally exist in relatively low levels in fish scattered around the oceans, can run rampant in densely packed fish farms.

The problems of animal wastes are a natural consequence of raising so many animals for food. The volume produced is so large that it is straining the environment and building to the point where future catastrophes are inevitable.

It's Getting Hot in Here!

Another problem associated with animal agriculture is the production of greenhouse gases. These gases trap heat in the earth's atmosphere and contribute to warming up the planet. Global warming is currently the focus of intense concern by environmental scientists.

According to a recent report published by the United Nations Food and Agriculture Organization, the livestock sector generates more greenhouse gas emissions, as measured in CO2 equivalent, than the transportation industry. (Note: Some greenhouse gases are more powerful than others. For example, methane is 21 times more effective than carbon dioxide at heating the atmosphere. Greenhouse gas emissions are often calculated in terms of how much CO2 would be needed to produce a similar warming effect. This is called "CO2 equivalent.") That's more emissions than all the cars, trucks, trains, ships, and airplanes put together. Remember that the production of food from animals uses most of the fossil fuel in American agriculture. When fossil fuel is burned, carbon dioxide is emitted. Carbon dioxide is a familiar greenhouse gas, but there are other greenhouse gases as well. Methane is important because it is more powerful as a greenhouse gas than carbon dioxide. Methane is produced in the animal waste lagoons mentioned earlier in this chapter. It is also produced in the stomachs and intestines of farm animals. As you can see in Table 6.3, livestock and manure constitute a significant portion of methane emissions. Equally important are nitrogen oxides, which also come from animal wastes.

A switch to a vegetarian diet would reduce greenhouse emissions by 3,267 pounds per person per year. Now consider that there are 300 million Americans. If we all went vegetarian, we would reduce American greenhouse emissions by about 980 billion pounds per year!

Here Today, Gone Tomorrow

> *It doesn't take man long to use up a continent.*
> —Robert Frost

Consider the effect that raising meat has on some of the world's ecosystems. Soil erosion is a significant ecological concern. One measure of a country's wealth is the quality and quantity of its soil, since this determines agricultural output. Soil doesn't appear overnight. It typically takes about 250

Percentage of Methane Produced by Human Activity
(Table 6.3)

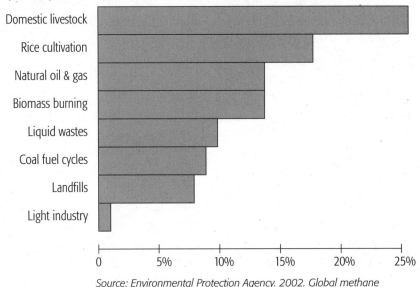

Source: *Environmental Protection Agency. 2002. Global methane emissions caused by human activity.*

years to produce one inch of farm soil. With this in mind, the importance of soil conservation becomes clear.

Unfortunately, raising cattle is the primary cause of soil erosion in the United States today; livestock grazing accounts for 85 percent of topsoil loss. Obviously, this has serious implications for American agriculture.

Many people are concerned about the growth of the world's deserts. It is important to recognize that the most significant cause of desertification in dry and semidry regions is overgrazing by too many livestock. According to the Council on Environmental Quality, overgrazing has been the most potent force behind desertification, in terms of the total acreage affected, within the United States. Not only an American problem, desertification is being experienced in places like China, where the Gobi Desert is overtaking what was once productive agricultural land, and in sub-Saharan Africa, where desertification is a major factor in famine.

There has been a catastrophic clearing of the Amazonian and Central American rain forests which has largely been done to create grazing land so that cattle can be raised for export, primarily to European markets. According to the Center for International Forestry Research, beef exports have accelerated the destruction of the Amazon rain forest. The total area destroyed increased from 102.5 million acres in 1990 to 145 million acres in 2000. In only 10 years, an area twice the size of Portugal was destroyed, almost all of it to clear pasture for cattle. David Kaimowitz, Director of the Center for International Forestry Research, says, "Cattle ranchers are making mincemeat out of Brazil's rain forests."

The rain forest is home to a large number of animals and plants, including many rare and endangered species that are being destroyed by cattle ranching. Almost as bad is the fact that tropical rain forest land cleared for pasture is very susceptible to soil erosion, given the special nature of rain forest soil and the special climate in tropical regions. Switching to a vegetarian diet would go a long way in helping to preserve tropical rain forests.

Your Environmental Footprint

Food is more than just a meal; it is a major industrial endeavor of mankind. Raising animals for food wastes water, grain, and oil, and causes massive ecological destruction, just to produce a product that is much less nutritious than vegetarian alternatives.

We all walk on the earth and can't help but leave a footprint. Following a vegetarian diet is a way of walking more softly on the earth. Leaving a smaller footprint not only sustains the environment right now, it helps preserve it for future generations. As I often say, "Walk softly and carry a big black bean burrito!"

Chapter 7

Saving the Animals with Every Bite

Many people love and care about animals, and we all enjoy the good feeling that comes from caring for a newfound friend. We all find the thought of eating a cat or a dog repugnant. But are farm animals really any less worthy of our love and care? Just as with cats and dogs, farm animals are sensitive to pain and want to live full, contented lives. The way to show you care about farm animals is simply to follow a nutritious vegetarian diet. Every time you choose a veggie burger rather than a meat burger, for instance, you take a big step toward saving the life of a gentle cow.

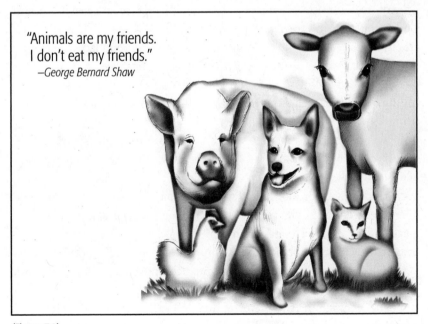

"Animals are my friends.
I don't eat my friends."
—*George Bernard Shaw*

(Figure 7.1)

Farm animals today are forced to live a much harder life than in former times. This is because the interests of modern factory farms revolve only around efficient, low-cost production, and unfortunately that results in greatly increased suffering for billions of animals. With growing public awareness of the increasingly inhumane conditions endured by today's farm animals, many people are questioning the treatment of these innocent creatures.

If you care about these animals and value their lives, you're not alone. In an Associated Press poll, two-thirds of Americans said that an animal's right to live free of suffering is just as important as a person's. Another third said that the existing laws are inadequate to protect animals. Worrying that animals are being treated inhumanely is a mainstream concern.

Caring about animals is as American as apple pie. Concern for our animal friends reaches across almost all demographic boundaries, and finds unlikely partners among congressmen and senators from both parties. Throughout history, statesmen and founding fathers have felt compassion for animals. William Penn, founder of the state of Pennsylvania, said "It is a cruel folly to offer up to ostentation so many lives of creatures as make up the state of our treats."

Thomas Paine, who started the American Revolution, said, "The moral duty of man consists of imitating the moral goodness and beneficence of God manifested in the creation, toward all his creatures....Everything of cruelty to animals is a violation of moral duty." Founding father Benjamin Franklin termed the eating of meat "unprovoked murder." But it was the great American president Abraham Lincoln who said it best: "I am in favor of animal rights as well as human rights. That is the way of a whole human being."

The vital concern about the suffering of farm animals also spans the centuries. Plato, Plutarch, Diogenes, Pythagoras, Ovid, and Seneca are just a few of the early philosophers who spoke out against the inherent cruelty involved in raising animals for food. The Renaissance artist, designer, inventor, and scientist Leonardo da Vinci said, "I have from an early age abjured the use of meat, and the time will come when men such as I will look upon the murder of animals as they now look upon the murder of men." More recently, actress Mary Tyler Moore also made a similar prediction: "It may take a while, but there will probably come a time when we look back and say, 'Good Lord, do you believe that in the twentieth century and early part of the twenty-first, people were still eating animals?'"

Some of America's greatest thinkers and writers have shown concern for the animals. Henry David Thoreau said, "I have no doubt that it is a part of the destiny of the human race, in its gradual improvement, to leave off eating animals."

No animal can write poetry or build a spaceship to the moon. But animals do share some critical attributes with humans—we both sense fear and we both feel pain. In 1789, English jurist, philosopher, and legal and social reformer Jeremy Bentham wrote, "The question is not, Can they [the animals] reason? nor, Can they talk? but, Can they suffer?" The obvious answer to anyone who thinks about the issue is yes.

The questions we are faced with are these: Is it humane to eat an animal raised in misery on a factory farm and killed in horrible circumstance in a slaughterhouse? Is it worthy of us as intelligent and sensitive human beings, as God's children?

That little round hamburger on a bun, smothered in ketchup and onions, gives few clues as to just how it came to be. Placed in a Styrofoam tray and wrapped in cellophane, that steak gives little indication that it was once a living, breathing, and feeling cow. Ralph Waldo Emerson expresses this predicament in the following way: "You have just dined, and however scrupulously the slaughterhouse is concealed in the graceful distance of miles, there is complicity."

In the olden days, a cow spent her life in the family farm's pasture. After many years of service, Grandpa would lead old Daisy behind the barn, take out his rifle, and it was over in a second. But it's not like that anymore. One needn't go into all the gory details, but a few samples must be digested to get the full picture. There is no better summary of the inhumane disaster taking place on America's factory farms than the description given by Senator Robert Byrd to the United States Senate (bear in mind that he was once a farmer):

"Our inhumane treatment of livestock is becoming widespread and more and more barbaric. Six-hundred-pound hogs—they were 'pigs' once—raised in two-foot-wide metal cages called gestational crates, in which poor beasts are unable to turn around or lie down in natural positions, and this is the way they live for months at a time.

On profit-driven factory farms, veal calves are confined to dark wooden crates so small they are prevented from lying down or scratching themselves. These creatures feel; they know pain. They suffer pain just as we humans suffer pain. Egg-laying hens are confined to battery cages [cages literally

115

stuffed so tight with chickens that they can barely move, and the cages are stacked on top of each other so that the wastes from the cages above fall on the chickens below]. Unable to spread their wings, they are reduced to nothing more than an egg-laying machine."

Battery-caged Hens (Figure 7.2)

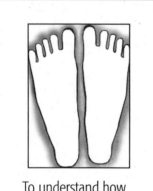

To understand how a battery hen lives, stand here for a year.

While compassion for animals is as American as apple pie, the situation on today's factory farms is rotten to the core. Even with broad-based American support, even with the support of several influential congressmen and senators, even with the support of a wide range of religious leaders from Pope John Paul II to the Dalai Lama, and even with the guidance of our founding fathers and other influential men and women throughout American history, the situation on the farms and in the slaughterhouses remains a nightmare and a national disgrace.

Most of us were taught to believe that milk production does not actually harm the cow, but this is no longer true. Dairy cows are forced to give birth repeatedly so that they can continuously produce milk. In many cases, they are injected with recombinant bovine growth hormone (rBGH), which is designed to produce an abnormally high volume of milk. This overproduction continually leads to mastitis and lameness, both painful afflictions. Dairy cows are raised to spend their lives producing milk only for human consumption, and when their milk production wanes after about three or four years, they are rounded up and sent to slaughter.

Scientists have determined that even fish are capable of suffering; unfortunately, fish are not the only animals hurt by the fishing industry. Modern fishing methods use very long nets to catch fish. Sea mammals such as dolphins, porpoises, and seals are also trapped in these nets and become casualties.

Although the current situation is dismal, to say the least, there is a hint of progress. California has become the first state to ban the production of foie gras. "Foie gras," French for "fat liver," is produced by force-feeding ducks and geese nearly to the point of explosion. And Florida became the first state to outlaw gestational crates for sows.

No one ever became a meat eater after a trip to a garden, but several people have become vegetarians after visiting a slaughterhouse. It has often been said that if slaughterhouses had glass walls, we would all be vegetarians. William F. Buckley Jr. agrees and made the following prediction, "When they notice what happens in abattoirs [slaughterhouses], there will be a serious movement against the eating of meat"

People are starting to notice, and this is one of the many reasons more and more people are adopting a vegetarian diet. Indeed, a vegetarian diet is considered by many to be the most effective way that people can express their natural compassion for other animals. In light of the fact that a vegetarian diet saves animals with every bite, many people say that the food not only tastes good but feels good as well. Of course, it should also be pointed out that the best way for us to reach old age is to help farm animals to do the same. A vegetarian diet lets everybody win.

Saving farm animals is easy. All you need to do is to make compassionate choices when shopping at the grocery store. Enjoy the many plant-based alternatives to meat, dairy, and eggs, and you too will be saving farm animals with every bite.

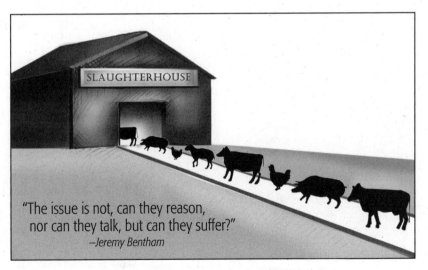

"The issue is not, can they reason, nor can they talk, but can they suffer?"
—Jeremy Bentham

(Figure 7.3)

Chapter 8

Food and Faith

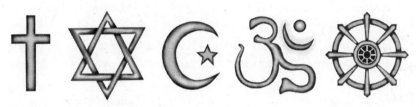

Whatever religious or spiritual path you follow, a vegetarian diet is a perfect fit! The world's religions have always recognized the spiritual importance of our food. Let's survey some of the world's religions and learn what they offer in support of a vegetarian diet.

In the Jewish religion there are the following principles: saving human life and health, not causing suffering to animals, feeding the hungry, and not wasting resources or harming the environment. All have a very solid foundation in the Bible. The original diet in Genesis was vegetarian. The Book of Prophets tells us that our diet will be vegetarian in the end of times. In the Book of Proverbs, we are taught that the righteous man regards the life of his animals. In the Book of Daniel, we see the healthfulness of a vegetarian diet over one with meat. The Talmud states, "Kashrut teaches first of all that eating meat is itself a moral compromise.... Man ideally should not eat meat, for to eat meat a life must be taken, an animal must be put to death.... The Torah teaches a lesson in moral conduct, that man shall not eat meat unless he has a special craving for it, and shall eat it only occasionally and sparingly."

Many famous Jews throughout history have been vegetarians. Maimonides, one of the most influential rabbis in history, advocated a vegetarian diet. More recently, the first Chief Rabbi of the modern state of Israel, Abraham Isaac Kook Ha Kohane, and the late Shlomo Goren, a Chief Rabbi of Israel, both followed a vegetarian diet. The famous Jewish philosopher Martin Buber and the Jewish scientist and philosopher Albert Einstein were also vegetarians. Israel is said to have the second highest per capita rate of vegetarians in the world.

The Roman Catholic Church has also shown its belief in the spiritual value of vegetarianism. There are four Catholic orders that have followed a vegetarian diet: the Trappist, Benedictine, Franciscan, and Carthusian orders have all traditionally followed a vegetarian diet. Ron Pickarski, a Franciscan monk, has written one of the most popular vegetarian cookbooks on the market, including *Friendly Foods*. Brother Victor-Antoine d'Avila-Latourette, a Benedictine, has written two excellent vegetarian cookbooks: *This Good Food* and *From a Monastery Kitchen*. Looking beyond our personal well-being, Pope John Paul II said, "Respect for life and for the dignity of the human person also extends to the rest of creation." St. Francis of Assisi, known for his love and compassion for animals, said, "All things of creation are children of the Father and thus brothers of man.... Not to hurt our humble brethren is our first duty to them." Cardinal Newman similarly said, "Cruelty to animals is as if man did not love God." These three great Roman Catholics show through their words the spiritual importance of values that are reflected by following a vegetarian diet.

From the Protestant community we have such figures as John Wesley, the founder of the Methodist church, who said, "Thanks be to God, since I gave up flesh and wine I have been delivered from all physical ills." The founder of the Salvation Army, General Booth, also a vegetarian, said "God disapproves of all cruelty, whether to man or beast." He credited his vegetarian diet for all his energy and vigor. When asked where he got his energy, he said, "I owe it to my careful vegetarian diet." One of the other church leaders, Colonel Moss, obtained vegetarian recipes to publish in the Salvation Army journals.

The Seventh-day Adventist Church has been a leading advocate of a vegetarian diet for well over a hundred years. In addition to the scriptures mentioned previously, Adventists also take note of the following: "Know ye not that ye are the temple of God...." (1 Corinthians 3:16–17) "Beloved, I wish above all things that thou mayest prosper in health, even as thy soul prospereth." (III John 1:2) Ellen G. White, one of the founders of the Seventh-day Adventist Church, advocated a vegetarian diet in several books and publications. She said, "Vegetables, fruits, and grains should compose our diet. Not an ounce of flesh meat should enter our stomachs. The eating of flesh is unnatural. We are to return to God's original purpose in the creation of man." Approximately 55 percent of the members of the Seventh-day Adventist Church are vegetarians.

Reverend Andrew Linzey of the Church of England, professor of theology at the University of Nottingham, England, and research fellow at Oxford University, writes, "Vegetarianism can arguably claim to have the strongest Biblical support."

Reverend Alvin Van Pelt Hart, Episcopalian priest and chaplain of St. Luke's Hospital, says "We now have scientific evidence that vegetarianism is good for the body. The greatest spiritual teachers have always known that it is good for the soul."

In Section 89 of the book *Doctrine and Covenants,* written by Joseph Smith, founder of the Church of Jesus Christ of Latter-day Saints, we find the following statement, "Flesh of the beasts and also the fowls...they are to be used sparingly...and these God hath made for the use of man only in times of famine and excess of hunger." While not expressly forbidding the consumption of meat, the passage certainly seems to require exceptional circumstances for its use. Brigham Young said, "When men live to the age of a tree, their food will be fruit." Ezra Taft Benson, thirteenth President of the Mormon Church, said, "We need a generation of young people who, as Daniel, eat in a more healthy manner than to fare on the 'king's meat,' and whose countenances show it. But what needs additional emphasis are the positive aspects...the need for vegetables, fruits, and grain, particularly wheat.... We need a generation of people who eat in a healthier manner. In general, the more food we eat in its natural state and the less it is refined without additives, the healthier it will be for us."

The four Fillmores, founders of the Unity Church, actively advocated the practice of vegetarianism during their lifetimes, beginning with Charles Fillmore's original article "As To Meat Eating," published in the October 1903 issue of *Unity Magazine.* Lowell Fillmore added the "New Thought Diet" section to *Unity Magazine* in 1906, and there were two special vegetarian issues of the magazine in February 1911 and June 1915. John Fillmore was editor of "The Vegetarian" column, which was added to *Weekly Unity* beginning with the October 25, 1911, issue.

Many early Quakers are said to have followed a vegetarian diet, consistent with their belief in universal compassion. The famous Quaker John Woolman said, "To say we love God as unseen and at the same time exercise cruelty towards the least creature moving by his life or by life derived from him is a contradiction in itself."

According to *Science and Health with Key to the Scriptures*, a major scripture of Christian Science, "God is the life or intelligence which forms and preserves the individuality and identity of animals as well as of man." *The Christian Science Journal* has also contained articles advocating a vegetarian diet.

A religion in the UK with a small but important following, the Order of the Cross, teaches pacifism and nonviolence to living beings. It requires their members to follow a vegetarian diet.

Dexter Scott King, son of Dr. Martin Luther King, Jr. and a vegan, said "Veganism has given me a higher level of awareness and spirituality." Noted Christian theologian, medical missionary, and vegetarian Albert Schweitzer said, "Until we extend the circle of compassion to all living things, humanity will not find peace."

Sylvester Graham was an American Presbyterian minister (ordained in 1826) who advocated a vegetarian diet. He was known for inventing the graham cracker. His *Graham Journal of Health and Longevity* preached his principles of good health, especially through a vegetarian diet.

Islam does not require the adoption of a vegetarian diet, but an argument can be made that the current treatment of farm animals would violate the prophet Muhammad's teachings. David Samuel Margoliouth, one of Muhammad's chief biographers, writes, "His humanity extended itself to the lower creation. . . . Acts of cruelty were swept away by him." Abu Hamid al-Ghazali, one of Islam's most brilliant philosophers, states in his book *Ihya Ulum ul Din*, "Compassionate eating leads to compassionate living." The Hunza tribe, living in northern Pakistan in the foothills of the Himalayas, follows a nearly vegetarian diet. They are famous for their longevity, often living to the age of 100, and are frequently thought of as the healthiest people in the world. They have been following a largely vegetarian diet for hundreds of years and give proof to the hadith, or popular saying of the prophet Muhammad, that "whoever is kind to one of God's creatures is kind to himself."

In the Buddhist religion, transmigration of the soul allows for animals to be past or future human beings. Therefore the killing and eating of animals is discouraged. This doctrine of karma discourages the killing and eating of animals, as doing so violates the principle of ahimsa, which means "nonviolence." The Mahaparinirvana Sutra states, "Whoever consumes meat extinguishes the seed of compassion." Buddha himself is said to have been vegetarian. It is no surprise that many of his followers also choose not to eat meat.

The Dalai Lama advocates a vegetarian diet, saying, "I do not see any reason why animals should be slaughtered to serve as human diet when there are so many substitutes. After all, man can live without meat.... There is no justification in indulging in such acts of brutality.... Still, the best way is to be vegetarian."

In China and Japan, many Buddhists are particularly careful about observing a vegetarian diet. Most notable among the many Chan Buddhists of China is Chu-hung, who very actively promoted vegetarianism. In Seattle and in other parts of the United States, you will find vegetarian restaurants operated by Chinese Buddhists. In his book *The Chain of Compassion,* the famous Japanese Zen master D. T. Suzuki says, "Buddhists must strive to teach respect and compassion for all creation—compassion is the foundation of their religion."

Confucius was a vegetarian, and many scholars believe that he introduced chopsticks in China so as to be able to eat without utensils that would remind him of the slaughterhouse.

The Hindu religion, which predates Buddhism, shares with it the concepts of karma and ahimsa and is famous for promoting vegetarianism. Perhaps one of the most famous vegetarians in recent times is Mahatma Gandhi, who said, "I do feel that spiritual progress does demand at some stage that we should cease to kill our fellow creatures." In the Vedic scriptures there are many passages that support vegetarianism. One passage states, "Having well considered the origin of flesh foods, and the cruelty of fettering and slaying corporeal beings, let man entirely abstain from eating flesh." Emphasizing the Hindu conception of the unity of all life, Srila Prabhupada, founder of the International Society for Krishna Consciousness, said, "Everyone is God's creature, although in different bodies or dresses. God is considered the one supreme father. A father may have many children, and some may be intelligent and others not very intelligent, but if an intelligent son tells his father, 'my brother is not very intelligent; let me kill him,' will the father agree? Similarly, if God is the supreme Father, why should He sanction the killing of animals who are also His sons?"

In the Sikh religion, originating in India, the Namdari sect and the Bahjan Golden Temple movement are strictly vegetarian. According to Sikh scholar Swaran Singh Sanehi, "Sikh scriptures support vegetarianism fully." The Jain religion, also originating in India, follows the ahimsa principle quite strictly. The Jains are famous for their devotion to and advocacy of vegetarianism.

Following a vegetarian diet has long been supported by many of the world's spiritual traditions. Dating back thousands of years in some cases, people of many different faiths have found a vegetarian diet an important part of their spiritual beliefs and practices. As time moves forward, more and more people are being inspired to adopt a vegetarian diet.

Afterword

By now you have come to understand the importance of our food choices. They occupy a central position in our world by exercising a profound effect on the environment, on the animals who inhabit the earth, on the world's hungry and, perhaps most profoundly, on the health and length of our own lives. When we choose to follow a healthy vegetarian diet we have taken a powerful step to improve our lives and the world we live in.

More than just a meal, the food we eat connects us with other members of our community starting with the farmer and ending in the kitchen, with so many hard working people in between. More and more people are turning to a vegetarian diet and the sales of healthful vegetarian foods have been growing quickly. Sensing that vegetarian food is the wave of the future many large companies have started to develop a line of vegetarian products.

Modern medical researchers have started to intensively study vegetarians, switching their focus from one of caution to enthusiastic endorsement of their diet. Environmentalists are recognizing that the vegetarian diet was the missing piece of the puzzle for a sustainable lifestyle. Our country as a whole is coming to realize that farm animals are living, feeling beings capable of suffering and deserving of something more natural than the factory farm. Furthermore, a growing number of religious leaders are recommending following a vegetarian diet as a laudable choice.

The vegetarian diet is an idea whose time has come. This book is just a beginning. The references will provide you with the necessary information to learn even more.

I wish all of you healthy lives in a healthy world.

Stewart Rose

May 17, 2007

Vegetarians of Washington

Something special is happening in the state of Washington. A new kind vegetarian society, Vegetarians of Washington, is growing by leaps and bounds and now has a membership numbering in the thousands. Vegetarians of Washington, an independent 501(c)3 non-profit organization founded in 2001, is already the largest and most dynamic regional vegetarian society in the United States and has the most enthusiastic and devoted members and supporters anywhere.

What makes Vegetarians of Washington so different? First is our membership. Vegetarians of Washington is made up of people from all walks of life. You don't even have to be a vegetarian to join! We don't ask and we don't tell. We welcome everyone whether they're an experienced vegetarian, a beginner or just curious.

Second is our approach. Vegetarians of Washington follows the education and advocacy model. We teach, we encourage and we try to have as much fun as we can while we do it. We're not activists. We don't hit people over the head with the tofu. Instead, we believe in providing a "can do" atmosphere where everybody proceeds at their own pace and just does the best they can, when changing over to a vegetarian diet.

Third are our events. We enjoy great tasting food and will accept nothing less. We hold gourmet monthly dining events at the Mount Baker Club in Seattle, where you can enjoy a delicious multi-course meal from a different local restaurant, chef or cookbook author each month, and meet lots of interesting people at one convenient location. We also hold free informative nutrition and cooking classes at locations throughout western Washington.

Our biggest event, Vegfest, held in March of each year in Seattle, Washington, is the largest vegetarian food festival in the United States. Vegfest features over 600 different kinds of food to try, talks on health and nutrition by doctors and dieticians, cooking demonstrations by chefs and cookbook authors, a huge vegetarian bookstore and a special children's program. Vegfest is attended by thousands of people and is staffed by over 700 volunteers who serve over 500,000 samples of food each year.

Fourth are our benefits. Our members receive a free subscription to the popular Vegetarian Times magazine. This unique magazine is packed full of recipes and the latest nutritional information. Our discount program entitles members to discounts at local restaurants and a wide range of businesses. Members also receive a reduced price at our dinners and special member's appreciation events.

Fifth are our books. *The Vegetarian Solution* is the latest book project of the Vegetarians of Washington, and the organization has devoted considerable time and effort to its production. We have written two books prior to this. The first is a guidebook to vegetarian dining, shopping and living in Washington and Oregon, called *Veg-Feasting in the Pacific Northwest*. The second is *The Veg-Feasting Cookbook* where we invited many local veg-friendly restaurants and chefs to share their very best recipes. All three books are currently available in fine bookstores everywhere or online.

Sixth is our work with vegetarian and veg-friendly businesses. Manufacturers, distributors and retailers of vegetarian foods and vegetarian restaurants form the vital links in our food chain. We work in many capacities to support those who bring us the food we eat thus closing the circle between producers and consumers.

Many wonderful people have joined Vegetarians of Washington. We meet their needs by creating a positive atmosphere where they can socialize, have fun, eat great food together, and reinforce their excellent choice to follow a vegetarian diet. Please join us! For more information, please visit us on the Web at www.VegOfWA.org or give us a call at 206 706 2635. To join, visit www.VegOfWA.org/joinus.html

Vegetarians of Washington
www.VegOfWA.org
206 706 2635

References

Many hours of research went into producing this book. The book is fully referenced. In order to increase its readability, we've chosen to leave out the footnote numbering. The references listed here are just a small fraction of the research that is available. Where only one study is referenced, this does not mean that only one study has found these results. There were many other studies which were not referenced due to space constraints.

Chapter 1—Introduction

It's Natural

Collins, William S. 1969. Atherosclerotic Disease: an Anthropologic Theory. *Medical Counterpoint* 12:54-55

Mills, Milton. 2006. The Comparative Anatomy of Eating. www.geocities.com/Rainforest/2062/ana.html

It's Healthy

American Dietetic Association. 2003. Position of the American Dietetic Association and dietitians of Canada: Vegetarian Diets. *Journal of the American Dietetic Association* 103(6):748-766

Barnard, Neal. 1995. *Eat Right Live Longer.* Three Rivers Press

Chang-Claude, Jenny, Rainer Frentzel-Beyme and Ursula Eilber. 1992. Mortality Pattern of German Vegetarians after 11 years of follow-up. *Epidemiology* 3(5):395-401

Fraser, Gary E. 1999. Associations between diet and cancer, ischemic heart disease, and all-cause mortablity in non-Hispanic white California Seventh-day Adventists. *American Journal of Clinical Nutrition* 70(3):532S-538S

Fraser, Gary E, and D.F. Shavlik. 2001. Ten years of life: Is it a matter of choice? *Archives of Internal Medicine* 161(13):1645-52

Fuhrman, Joel. 2003. *Eat to Live.* New York: Little, Brown and Company

Jenkins, David J.A. et al. 2005. Direct Comparison of a dietary portfolio of cholesterol-lowering foods with a statin in hypercholesterolemic participants. *American Journal of Clinical Nutrition* 81(2):380-387

Krajcovicova-Kudlackova, M. 1995. Selected vitamins and trace elements in blood of vegetarians. *Annals of Nutrition and Metabolism* 39(6):334-9

Margetts, Barrie M. and Alan A. Jackson. 1993. Vegetarians and Longevity – letter to the Editor. *Epidemiology* 4(3):278-279

McCarty, M.F. 2003. A low-fat, whole-food vegan diet, as well as other strategies that down-regulate IGF-I activity, may slow the human aging process. *Medical Hypotheses* 60(6):784-92

McKevith, B. 2005. Diet and healthy aging. *Journal of the British Menopause Society* 11(4):121-5

McMichael, Anthony J. 1992. Vegetarians and Longevity: Imagining a Wider Reference Population, *Epidemiology* 3(5):389-391

Messina, V. and K. Burke. 1997. Position on Vegetarian Diets. *Journal of the American Dietetic Association* 97:1317-21

Ornish, Dean et al. 1998. Intensive Lifestyle Changes for Reversal of Coronary Heart Disease. *Journal of American Medical Association* 280:2001-2007

Singh, Pramil N., Joan Sabate and Gary Fraser. 2003. Does low meat consumption increase life expectancy in humans? *American Journal of Clinical Nutrition* 78 (Suppl):526S-532S

Richter, V. and F. Rassoul. 2004. Ageing, cardiovascular risk profile and vegetarian nutrition. *Asia Pacific Journal of Clinical Nutrition* 13(Suppl):S107

Segasothy, M. and Phillips P.A. 1999. Vegetarian diet: panacea for modern lifestyle diseases? *Quarterly Journal of Medicine* 92(9):531-544

Snowdon, David A. 1988. Animal product consumption and mortality because of all causes combined, coronary heart disease, stroke, diabetes, and cancer in Seventh-day Adventists. *American Journal of Clinical Nutrition* 48:739-48

It's Easy

Barnard, Neal and Andrew Nicholson. 1995. The medical costs attributable to meat consumption. *Preventative Medicine* 24, 646-655

Lea, E.J. et al. 2005. Consumers' readiness to eat a plant-based diet. *European Journal of Clinical Nutrition* 60:342-351

Moore Lappé, Frances. 1991. *Diet for a Small Planet 20th Anniversary Edition.* New York: Ballantine Books

Ornish, Dean. 1996. *Reversing Heart Disease.* New York: Ivy Books

It's Popular

Giehl, Dudley. 1979. *Vegetarianism.* New York: Harper and Row

Gregerson, Jon. 1994. *Vegetarianism A History.* Fremont, CA: Jain Publishing Co.

Iacobbo, Karen and Michael. 2006. *Vegetarians and Vegans in America Today.* Praeger

Iacobbo, Karen and Michael. 2004. *Vegetarian America.* Praeger

Chapter 2 - Moving Toward a Vegetarian Diet

Redmond, Cheryl. 2005. The Vegetarian Kitchen in *The Veg-Feasting Cookbook.* Vegetarians of Washington, Book Publishing Company

Chapter 3 – A Diet for all Ages

Pregnancy and Infancy

Dagnelie, P.C. et al. 1992. Nutrients and contaminants in human milk from mothers on macrobiotic and omnivorous diets. *European Journal of Clinical Nutrition* 46(5):355-66

Dorea, Jose G. 2004. Vegetarian diets and exposure to organochlorine pollutants, lead, and mercury. *American Journal of Clinical Nutrition* 80(1): 237-238

Hergenrather, Jeffrey et al. 1981. Pollutants in Breast Milk of Vegetarians. *New England Journal of Medicine* 304(13):792

Huncharek, M. and B. Kupelnick. 2004. A meta-analysis of maternal cured meat consumption during pregnancy and the risk of childhood brain tumors. *Neuroepidemiology* 23(1-2):78-84

Kannan, K. et al. 1997. Organochlorine pesticides and polychlorinated biphenyls in foodstuffs from Asian and Oceanic countries. *Reviews of Environmental Contamination and Toxicology* 152:1-55

Merritt, Russell J. and Belinda H. Jenks. 2004. Safety of Soy-based Infant Formulas Containing Isoflavones: The Clinical Evidence. *Journal of Nutrition* 134:1220S-1224S

Messina, V. and K. Burke. 1997. The American Dietetic Association Position on Vegetarian Diets. *Journal of the American Dietetic Assoc.* 97:1317-21

Noren, K. 1983. Levels of organochlorine contaminants in human milk in relation to the dietary habits of the mothers. *Acta Paediatrica Scandinavica* 72(6):811-6

Schecter, Arnold et al. 2001. Intake of Dioxins and Related Compounds from Food in the US Population. *Journal of Toxicology and Environmental Health Part A,* 63:1-18

Smith, Kimberly M. and Nadine R. Sahyoun. 2005. Fish consumption: recommendations versus advisories, can they be reconciled? *Nutrition Reviews* 63(2):39-46

Tsukino, H. et al. 2006. Fish Intake and serum levels of organochlorines among Japanese women. *The Science of the Total Environment* 359(1-3):90-100

van Kaam, A.H. et al. 1991. Polychlorobiphenyls in human milk, adipose tissue, plasma and umbilical cord blood; levels and correlates (article in Dutch). *Ned Tijdschr Geneeskd* 3;135(31):1399-403

Healthy Children

Dwyer, J.T. et al. 1980. Mental age and I.Q. of predominantly vegetarian children. *Journal of the American Dietetic Assoc.* 76(2):142-7

O'Connell, J.M. et al. 1989. Growth of vegetarian children: The Farm study. *Pediatrics* 84(3):475-81

Sabate, J. et al. 1991. Attained height of lacto-ovo vegetarian children and adolescents. *European Journal of Clinical Nutrition* 45:51-58

Type 1 Diabetes

Dahlquist, G. et al. 1992. An increased level of antibodies to beta-lactoglobulin is a risk determinant for early-onset type 1 (insulin-dependent) diabetes mellitus independent of islet cell antibodies and early introduction of cow's milk. *Diabetologia* 35(10):980-4

Paronen, Johanna et al. 2000. Effect of cow's milk exposure and maternal type 1 diabetes on cellular and humoral immunization to dietary insulin in infants at genetic risk for type 1 diabetes. *Diabetes* 49(10):1657-1665

Saukkonen, T. et al. 1998. Significance of cow's milk protein antibodies as risk factor for childhood IDDM: interactions with dietary cow's milk intake and HLA-DQB1 genotype. Childhood Diabetes in Finland Study Group. *Diabetologia* 41(1):72-78

Vaarala, O. et al. 1999. Cow's milk formula feeding induces primary immunization to insulin in infants at genetic risk for type 1 diabetes. *Diabetes* 48(7):1389-94

Cancer

Dietrich, M. et al. 2005. A review: Dietary & endogenously formed N-nitroso compounds and risk of childhood brain tumors. *Cancer Causes Control* 16(6):619-35

Jensen, C.D. et al. 2004. Maternal dietary risk factors in childhood acute lymphoblastic leukemia (United States). *Cancer Causes Control* 15(6):559-70

Peters, J.M. et al. 1994. Processed meats and risk of childhood leukemia (California, USA). *Cancer Causes Control* 5(2):195-202

Preston-Martin, S. et al. 1996. Maternal consumption of cured meats in relation to pediatric brain tumors. *Cancer Epidemiology Biomarkers and Prevention* 5(8):599-605

Sarasua, S. and D.A. Savitz. 1994. Cured and broiled meat consumption in relation to childhood cancer: Denver, Colorado (United States). *Cancer Causes Control* 5(2):141-8

The Teenage Years

Altman, Nathaniel. 1973. *Eating for Life*. The Theosophical Publishing House

Berenson G. et al. 1998. Association between multiple cardiovascular risk factors and atherosclerosis in children and young adults. *New England Journal of Medicine* 338:1650-1656

Collins, William S. 1969. Atherosclerotic Disease: an Anthropologic Theory. *Medical Counterpoint* 12:54-55

Enos, W.F., R.H. Holmes, and J. Beyer. 1953. Coronary disease among United States soldiers killed in action in Korea. *Journal of the American Medical Assoc.* 152:1090-1093

McMahan, C.A. et al. 2005. Risk Scores Predict Atherosclerotic Lesions in Young People. *Archives of Internal Medicine* 165:883-890

McNamara, J.J. et al. 1971. Coronary artery disease in combat casualties in Vietnam. *Journal of the American Medical Assoc.* 216:1185-1187

Strong, J.P. et al. 1999. Prevalence and extent of atherosclerosis in adolescents and young adults. *Journal of the American Medical Assoc.* 281:727-735

Zieske, A.W., G.T. Malcolm, and J.P. Strong. 2002. Natural history and risk factors in atherosclerosis in children and youth: the PDAY study. *Pediatric Pathology & Molecular Medicine* 21(2):213-37

Adebamowo, C.A. et al. 2005. High school dietary dairy intake and teenage acne. *Journal of American Academy of Dermatology* 52(2):207-215

Barnard, Neal D. et al. 2000. Diet and Sex-Hormone Binding Globulin, Dysmenorrhea and Premenstrual Symptoms. *Obstetrics & Gynecology* 95(2):245-250

Lanou, Amy Joy et al. 2005. Calcium, Dairy Products and Bone Health in Children and Young Adults: A Reevaluation of the Evidence. *Pediatrics* 115(3):736-743

Lindahl, O. et al. 1985. Vegan regimen with reduced medication in the treatment of bronchial asthma. *Journal of Asthma* 22(1):45-55

Stoll, B.A., L.J. Vatten and S. Kvinnsland. 1994. Does early physical maturity influence breast cancer risk? *Acta Oncologica* 33(2):171-6

Winning the Race on a Vegetarian Diet

Astrand, Per Olaf. 1968. *Nutrition Today* 3(2):9-11

Barr, Susan I. and Candice A. Rideout. 2004. Nutritional considerations for vegetarian athletes, *Nutrition* 20(7-8):696-703

Haub, M.D. et al. 2002. Effect of protein source on resistive-training-induced changes in body composition and muscle size in older men. *American Journal of Clinical Nutrition* 76(3):511-7

Jurek, Scott. 2004. Winning the race on a vegetarian diet in *Veg-Feasting in the Pacific Northwest,* Vegetarians of Washington, Book Publishing Company.

Nieman, David C. 1999. Physical fitness and vegetarian diets - is there a relation? *American Journal of Clinical Nutrition* 70(3):570S-573S

Pearl, Bill. 2001. *Getting Stronger* p 374, 429. Bolinas, CA: Shelter Publications.

Chapter 4 – Common Diseases

Introduction

Barnard, Neal and Andrew Nicholson. 1995. The medical costs attributable to meat consumption. *Preventative Medicine* 24:646-655

Brown, Lester R. 1995. *Who Will Feed China?* pg 46. New York: W.W. Norton & Company

Campbell, T. Colin. 2004. *The China Study.* Dallas Texas: Benbella Books

Key, Timothy and Gwyneth Davey. 1996. Prevalence of obesity is low in people who do not eat meat. *British Medical Journal* 313:816-817

Lampe, J.W. 1999. Health effects of vegetables and fruit: assessing mechanisms of action in human experimental studies. *American Journal of Clinical Nutrition* 70 (3-Suppl):475S-490S

Nelson, Ethel R. 1974. *375 Meatless Recipes.* Leominster Mass: Eussey Press

Nierenberg, Danielle. 2003. Meat production and consumption grow. *Vital Signs* pgs 30-31. Washington D.C.: World Watch Institute

Ornish, Dean. 1995. *Reversing Heart Disease.* New York: Ivy Books

Segasothy, M. and Phillips P.A. 1999. Vegetarian diet: panacea for modern lifestyle diseases? *Quarterly Journal of Medicine* 92(9):531-544

The Shifting Paradigm of Vegetarian Diets

Burkitt, Denis. 1991. An approach to the reduction of the most common Western cancers. *Archives of Surgery* 126(3):345-7

Esselstyn, Caldwell B. Jr. 1991. American Assoc of Endocrine Surgeons Presidential Address: Beyond Surgery. *Surgery* 110(6):923-7

Kennedy, E.T. 2006. Evidence for nutritional benefits in prolonging wellness. *American Journal of Clinical Nutrition* 83(2):410S-414S

McFarland, J. Wayne. 1974. Foreword *375 Meatless Recipes,* by Ethel Nelson. Leominster, Mass: Eussey Press

Nestle, Marion et al. 1998. Behavioral and Social Influences on Food Choice. *Nutrition Review* 56(5): (II)S50-S74

Ornish, Dean. 1995. *Reversing Heart Disease.* New York: Ivy Books

Sabate, Joan. 2003. The contribution of vegetarian diets to health and disease: a paradigm shift? *American Journal of Clinical Nutrition* 78(3):502S-507S

Smith, R.E., B.R. Olin and J.W. Madsen. 2006. Spitting into the wind: the irony of treating chronic disease. *Journal of the American Pharmacists Assoc.* (Wash DC) 46(3):379-400

Getting to the Heart of the Matter

American Heart Association. 1995. Heart and Stroke Facts. *American Heart Association 1995 Statistical supplement*

Anderson, J.W. 1990. Serum lipid response of hypercholesterolemic men to single and divided doses of canned beans. *American Journal of Clinical Nutrition* 51(6):1013-9

Barnard, N.D. et al. 2004. Acceptability of a low-fat vegan diet compares favorably to a step II diet in a randomized, controlled trial. *Journal of Cardiopulmonary Rehabilitation* 24(4):229-35

Castelli, William P. 1984. Epidemiology of coronary heart disease. *American Journal of Medicine* 76:4-12

Castelli, William P. 1979. Letter, Oct 19. *National Institute of Health*

Cohen, Jonathan C., et al. 2006. Sequence variations in PCSK9, low LDL, and protection against coronary heart disease. *New England Journal of Medicine* 354:1264-1272

Demonty, Isabelle, Benoit Lamarche, and Peter J.H. Jones. 2003. Role of isoflavones in the hypocholesterolemic effect of soy. *Nutrition Reviews* 61(6):189-203

Editorial. 1961. *Journal of the American Medical Association,* 176(9):806

Esselstyn, Caldwell B. Jr. 2000. In cholesterol lowering, moderation kills. *Cleveland Clinic Journal of Medicine* 67(8):560-4

Flight, I. 2006. Cereal grains and legumes in the prevention of coronary heart disease and stroke: a review of the literature. *European Journal of Clinical Nutrition* 60, 1145–1159

Fraser, G.E., K.D. Lindsted and W.L. Beeson. 1995. Effect of risk factor values on lifetime risk of and age at first coronary event. The Adventist Health Study. *American Journal of Epidemiology* 142(7):746-758

Fraser, G.E. 1999. Associations between diet and cancer, ischemic heart disease and all cause mortality in Seventh Day Adventists in non-Hispanic white California Seventh Day Adventists. *American Journal of Clinical Nutrition* 70(3):532S-538S

Fraser, G.E. 1992. A possible protective effect of nut consumption on risk of coronary heart disease. The Adventist Health Study, *Archives of Internal Medicine* 152(7):1416-24

Fu, C.H., C.C. Yang, C.L. Lin and T.B. Kuo. 2006. Effects of long-term vegetarian diets on cardiovascular autonomic functions in healthy postmenopausal women. *American Journal of Cardiology.* 97(3):380-3

Gardner, Christopher D. et al. 2005. The effect of a plant-based diet on plasma lipids in hypercholesterolemic adults. *Annals of Internal Medicine* 142(9):725-733

Hu, Frank B. et al. 1998. Frequent nut consumption and risk of coronary heart disease in women. *British Medical Journal* 317:1341-1345

Hu, Frank B. 2003. Plant-based foods and prevention of cardiovascular disease: an overview. *American Journal of Clinical Nutrition* 78(3):544S-551S

Jenkins, David J.A. et al. 2005. Diet and Cholesterol Reduction. *Annals of Internal Medicine* 142:725-733

Kris-Etherton, Penny M. et al. 2001. The effect of nuts on coronary heart disease risk. *Nutrition Reviews* 59(4):103-111

National Heart, Lung and Blood Institute. 2006. www.nhlbi.nih.gov/actintime/aha.aha.htm

Ornish, Dean et al. 1998. Intensive lifestyle changes for reversal of coronary heart disease. *Journal of the American Medical Assoc.* 280:2001-2007

Ornish, Dean. 1995. *Reversing Heart Disease.* New York: Ivy Books

Rosell, Magdalena S. et al. 2004. Soy intake and blood cholesterol concentrations: a cross-sectional study of 1033 pre- and postmenopausal women in the Oxford arm of the European Prospective Investigation into Cancer and Nutrition. *American Journal of Clinical Nutrition* 80(5):1391-1396

Slavicek, J. et al (Czech). 2001. Effect of a 10-day animal fat-free diet on cholesterol and glucose serum levels, blood pressure and body weight in 50-yr old volunteers. *Sbornik Lekarsky* 102(4):519-25

Snowdon, D.A., R.L. Phillips and G.E. Fraser. 1984. Meat consumption and fatal ischemic heart disease. *Preventative Medicine* 13(5):490-500

Szeto, Y.T., T.C. Kwok and I.F. Benzie. 2004. Effects of a long-term vegetarian diet on biomarkers of antioxidant status and cardiovascular disease risk. *Nutrition* 20(10):863-6

Thorogood, M.et al. 1992. Plasma lipids and lipoprotein cholesterol conditions in people with different diets in Britain. *British Medical Journal* 295:351-353

No authors listed (article in Russian). 2005. The treatment of coronary heart disease by beta-adrenoblockers or tiazide diuretics preparation in combination with vegetarian diet. *Vopr Pitan* 74(3):39-41

Blood Pressure – Roll up your sleeve

Berkow, Susan E. and Neal D. Barnard. 2005. Blood pressure regulation and vegetarian diets. *Nutrition Reviews* 63(1):1-8

Goren, J.J. et al. 1962. The influence of nutrition and the ways of life on blood cholesterol and the prevalence of hypertension and coronary heart disease among Trappist and Benedictine Monks. *American Journal of Clinical Nutrition* 10:456-457

Moore, Thomas J. et al. 2001. DASH Diet is effective treatment for Stage 1 Isolated Systolic Hypertension. *Hypertension* 38:155

Moore, Thomas. 2001. *The Dash Diet for Hypertension.* New York: The Free Press

Rouse, I.L., B.K. Armstrong and L.J. Beilin. 1983. The relationship of blood pressure to diet and lifestyle of two religious populations. *Hypertension* 1:65-71

Sacks, F.M. and E.H. Kass. 1988. Low blood pressure in vegetarians: effects of specific foods and nutrients. *American Journal of Clinical Nutrition* 48:795-800

Stroke – All of a sudden...

Feldman, Elaine B. 2001. Fruits and vegetables and the risk of stroke. *Nutrition Reviews* 59(1):24-27

He, F.J., C.A. Nowson and G.A. MacGregor. 2006. Fruit and vegetable consumption and stroke: meta-analysis of cohort studies. *Lancet* 367(9507):320-6

Joshipura, Kaumudi J. et al. 1999. Fruit and vegetable intake in relation to risk of ischemic stroke. *Journal of the American Medical Assoc.* 282:1233-1239

Luc, Dauchet, Philippe Amouyel, and Jean Dallongeville. 2005. Fruit and vegetable consumption and risk of stroke - a meta-analysis of cohort studies. *Neurology* 65:1193-1197

Cancer

American Cancer Society, Cancer Facts and Figures 2004. www.cancer.org/docroot/STT/content/STT_1x_Cancer_Facts__Figures_2004.asp

Beecher, Gary R. 1999. Phytonutrients' role in metabolism: effects on resistance to degenerative processes. *Nutrition Reviews* 57(9): (II)S3-S6

Block, G., B. Patterson and A. Subar. 1992. Fruit, vegetables, and cancer prevention: a review of the epidemiological evidence. *Nutrition and Cancer* 18(1):1-29

Craig, Winston J. 2002. Phytochemicals: Guardians of our health. *Vegetarian Nutrition Updates,* March 12th, 2002

Doll, R., and R. Peto. 1981. The causes of cancer: quantitative estimates of avoidable risks of cancer in the United States today. *Journal of the National Cancer Institute* 66:1191-308

Gonzalez de Mejia, Elvira et al. 2003. The anticarcinogenic potential of soybean lectin and lunasin. *Nutrition Reviews* 61(7):239-246

Holmes, S. 2006. Nutrition and the prevention of cancer. *The Journal of Family Health Care* 16(2):43-6

Kannan, K. et al. 1997. Organochlorine pesticides and polychlorinated biphenyls in foodstuffs from Asian and Oceanic countries. *Reviews of Environmental Contamination & Toxicology* 152:1-55

Knize, Mark G. and James S. Felton. 2005. Formation and human risk of carcinogenic heterocyclic amines formed from natural precursors in meat. *Nutrition Reviews* 63(5):158-165

Lampe, J.W. 1999. Health effects of vegetables and fruit: assessing mechanisms of action in human experimental studies. *American Journal of Clinical Nutrition* 70 (3-Suppl):475S-490S

Lampe, Johanna W. 2003. Spicing up a vegetarian diet: chemopreventative effects of phytochemicals. *American Journal of Clinical Nutrition* 78(3):579S-583S

Rabin, B.M., B. Shukitt-Hale, J. Joseph and P. Todd. 2005. Diet as a factor in behavioral radiation protection following exposure to heavy particles. *Gravit Space Biol* Bull 18(2):71-7

Steinman, David. 1990. *Diet for a Poisoned Planet.* New York: Ballantine Books

Tao, M.H. et al. 2005. A case-control study in Shanghai of fruit and vegetable intake and endometrial cancer. *British Journal of Cancer* 92(11):2059-64

Tavani, A. and C. La Vecchia. 1995. Fruit and vegetable consumption and cancer risk in a Mediterranean population. *American Journal of Clinical Nutrition.* 61(6 Suppl):1374S-1377S

Breast Cancer

Awad, A.B., R. Roy, and C.S. Fink. 2003. Beta-sitosterol, a plant sterol, induces apoptosis and activated key caspases in MDA-MB-231 human breast cancer cells. *Oncology Reports* 10(2):497-500

Cho, Eunyoung et al. 2003. Premenopausal fat intake and risk of breast cancer. *Journal of National Cancer Institute.* 95(14):1079-85

de Stefani, E. et al. 1997. Meat intake, heterocyclic amines, and risk of breast cancer: a case-control study in Uruguay. *Cancer Epidemiology Biomarkers & Prevention* 6(8):573-581

Gaudet, Mia M. et al. 2004. Fruits, Vegetables and Micronutrients in Relation to Breast Cancer Modified by Menopause and Hormone Receptor Status. *Cancer Epidemiology Biomarkers & Prevention* 13:1485-1494

Hirayama, T. 1978. Epidemiology of breast cancer with special reference to the role of diet. *Preventative Medicine* 7(2):173-95

Hirose, K. et al. 2005. Soybean products and reduction of breast cancer risk: a case-control study in Japan. *British Journal of Cancer* 93(1):15-22

Holm, L.E., E. Nordevang et al. 1993. Treatment failure and dietary habits in women with breast cancer. *Journal of the National Cancer Institute* 85(10):32-36

Howe, G.R., T. Hirohata, T. Hislop, et al. 1990. Dietary factors and risk of breast cancer: combined analysis of 12 case-control studies. *Journal of the National Cancer Institute* 82:561-9

Jackson, Steven J.T. & Keith W. Singletary. 2004. Sulforaphane inhibits Human MCF-7 Mammary Cancer Cell Mitotic Progression and Tubulin Polymerization. *Journal of Nutrition* 134:2229-2236

McKeown, Nicola and Jean Mayer. 1999. Antioxidants and Breast Cancer. *Nutrition Reviews* 57(10):321-324

Rose, D.P., A.P. Boyer and A.L. Wynder. 1986. International Comparisons of Mortality for cancer of the breast, ovary and colon and per capita food consumption. *Cancer* 58 (11):2363-2371

Stoll, B.A. 1999. Western nutrition and the insulin resistance syndrome: a link to breast cancer. *European Journal of Clinical Nutrition* 53(2):83-7

Trichopoulou, A., et al. 1995. Consumption of olive oil and specific food groups in relation to breast cancer risk in Greece. *Journal of the National Cancer Institute* 87:110-16

Prostate Cancer

Chen, Y.C., et al. 2005. Diet, vegetarian food and prostate carcinoma among men in Taiwan. *British Journal of Cancer* 93:1057-1061

Giovannucci, E., et al. 1993. A prospective study of dietary fat and risk of prostate cancer. *Journal of the National Cancer Institute* 85(19):1571-9

Joseph, Michael A. et al. 2004. Cruciferous Vegetables, Genetic Polymorphisms in Glutathione, S-Transferases M1 and T1, and Prostate Cancer Risk. *Nutrition and Cancer* 50(2):206-213

Li-Qiang, Qin et al. 2004. Milk Consumption is a risk factor for Prostate Cancer: Meta-Analysis of Case-Control Studies. *Nutrition and Cancer* 48(1):22-27

McCann, S.E. 2005. Intakes of selected nutrients, foods, and phytochemicals and prostate cancer risk in western New York. *Nutrition and Cancer* 53(1):33-41

Messina, Mark J. 2003. Emerging Evidence on the Role of Soy in Reducing Prostate Cancer Risk. *Nutrition Reviews* 61(4):117-131

Ornish, D. et al. 2005. Intensive lifestyle changes may affect the progression of prostate cancer. *Journal of Urology* 174(3):1065-9

Prostate Cancer Foundation. 2006. www.prostatecancerfoundation.org

Shukla, S. and S. Gupta. 2005. Dietary agents in the chemoprevention of prostate cancer. *Nutrition and Cancer* 53(1):18-32

Sonn, G.A., W. Aronson, and M.S. Litwin. 2005. Impact of diet on prostate cancer: a review. *Prostate Cancer and Prostatic Diseases* 8(4):304-10

Thomas, John A. 1999. Diet, Micronutrients, and the Prostate Gland. *Nutrition Reviews* 57(4):95-103

Vij, U., and A. Kumar. 2004. Phyto-oestrogens and prostatic growth. *National Medical Journal of India* 17(1):22-6

Ovarian Cancer

Hanna, L. and M. Adams. 2006. Prevention of ovarian cancer. *Best Practice and Research Clinical Obstetrics and Gynaecology* 20(2):339-62

LaVecchia, C., A. DeCarli et al. 1987. Dietary factors and the risk of epithelial ovarian cancer. *Journal of the National Cancer Institute* 79(4):663-669

National Research Council. 1982. *Diet, Nutrition, and Cancer.* Washington, D.C.: National Academy Press

Lymphoma

Chiou, B.C., J.R. Cerhan et al. 1996. Diet and risk of Non-Hodgkin lymphoma in older women. *Journal of the American Medical Association* 275(17):1315-1321

Kelemen, L.E. et al. 2006. Vegetables, fruit, and antioxidant-related nutrients and risk of non-Hodgkin lymphoma: a National Cancer Institute-Surveillance, Epidemiology, and End Results population-based case-control study. *American Journal of Clinical Nutrition* 83(6):1401-10

Esophageal and Stomach Cancer

Brown, L., G. Swanson, G. Gridley et al. 1995. Adenocarcinoma of the esophagus: role of obesity and diet. *Journal of the National Cancer Institute* 87:104-109

Roth, Julie and Sohrad Mobarhan. 2001. Preventive Role of Dietary Fiber in Gastric Cardia Cancers. *Nutrition Reviews* 59(11):372-374

Terry, P., J. Lagergren, W. Ye et al. 2001. Inverse association between intake of cereal fiber and gastric cardia cancer. *Gastroenterology* 120:387-91

Zhang, Z., R. Kurtz, G. Yu et al. 1997. Adenocarcinoma of the esophagus and gastric cardia: the role of diet. *Nutrition and Cancer* 27:298-309

Pancreatic Cancer

Chan, J.M., F. Wang and E.A. Holly. 2005. Vegetable and fruit intake and pancreatic cancer in a population-based case-control study in the San Francisco bay area. *Cancer Epidemiology Biomarkers and Prevention* 14(9):2093-7

Colon Cancer

Bingham, S.A. et al. 2003. Dietary fibre in food and protection against colorectal cancer in the European Prospective Investigation into Cancer and Nutrition (EPIC): an observational study. *The Lancet* 361(9368):1496-501

Giovanucci E., MJ Stampfer et al. 1992. Relationship of diet to colorectal adenoma in men. *Journal of the National Cancer Institute* 84(2): 91-98

Howe, G.R., E. Benito et al. 1992. Dietary intake of fiber and decreased risk of cancers of the colon and rectum evidence of combined analysis of 13 case controlled studies. *Journal of the National Cancer Institute* 84(24):1887-1896

Le Marchand, Loic et al. 2002. Red Meat Intake, CYP2E1 Genetic Polymorphisms, and Colorectal Cancer Risk. *Cancer Epidemiology Biomarkers & Prevention* 11:1019-1024

Lewin, M.H. et al. 2006. Red meat enhances the colonic formation of the DNA adduct 06-carboxymethyl guanine: implications for colorectal cancer risk. *Cancer Research* 66(3):1859-65

Norat, Teresa and Elio Riboli. 2001. Meat Consumption and Colorectal Cancer: A Review of Epidemiologic Evidence. *Nutrition Reviews* 59(2):37-47

Steinmetz, K.A. and J.D. Potter. 1993. Food-group consumption and colon cancer in the Adelaide case – control study. II. Meat, poultry, seafood, dairy foods and eggs. *International Journal of Cancer* 53(5):720-727

Story, Jon A. and Dennis A. Savaiano. 2001. Dietary Fiber and Colorectal Cancer: What is Appropriate Advice? *Nutrition Reviews* 59(3):84-85

Willet, W.C., M.J. Stampher et al. 1990. Relation of meat fat and fiber intake to the risk of colon cancer among women. *New England Journal of Medicine* 323 (24):1664-1672

Lung Cancer

Brennan, P. et al. 2005. Effect of cruciferous vegetables on lung cancer in patients stratified by genetic status: a mendelian randomisation approach. *The Lancet* 366(9496):1558-60

Haughy, B.P., J.R. Marshall, et al. 1987. Diet and lung cancer risk: findings from the Western New York Diet Study. *American Journal of Epidemiology* 125(3):351-356

Hirayama, T. 1985. Mortality in Japanese with lifestyles similar to Seventh Day Adventists: Strategy for risk reduction by lifestyle modification. *National Cancer Institute Monograph* 69:143-145

Kellen, E. et al. 2006. Fruit consumption reduces the effect of smoking on bladder cancer risk. The Belgian case control study on bladder cancer. *International Journal of Cancer* 118(10):2572-8

Rylander, R. and G. Axelsson. 2006. Lung cancer risks in relation to vegetable and fruit consumption and smoking. *International Journal of Cancer* 118(3):739-43

Schabath, M.B. et al. 2005. Dietary phytoestrogens and lung cancer risk. *Journal of the American Medical Association* 294(12):1493-504

Obesity – Winning the Battle of the Bulge

Appleby, P.N. et al. 1998. Low body mass index in non-meat eaters: the possible roles of animal fat, dietary fibre and alcohol. *International Journal of Obesity and Related Metabolic Disorders* 22(5):454-60

Furhman Joel. 2003. *Eat to Live*. Little, Brown and Company, New York

Key, Timothy and Gwyneth Davey. 1996. Prevelence of obesity is low in people who do not eat meat. *British Medical Journal* 313:816-817

Laskowska-Klita, T. et al (article in Polish). 2004. Serum leptin concentration and some lipid parameters in vegetarian children. *Polski Merkuriusz Lekarski* 16(94):340-3

Medkova, I.L., L.I. Mosiakina and L.S. Biriukova (article in Russian). 2002. Estimation of action of lacto-ovo-vegetarian and vegan diets on blood level of atherogenic lipoproteins in healthy people. *Voprosy Pitaniia* 71(4):17-9

Newby, P.K., Katherine L. Tucker and Alicja Wolk. 2005. Risk of overweight and obesity among semivegetarian, lactovegetarian and vegan women. *American Journal of Clinical Nutrition* 81(6):1267-74

Phend, Crystal. 2006. *Obesity Epidemic Spreads to Infants* www.medpagetoday. com/Pediatrics/Obesity/tb/3907

Robinson, F. et al. 2002. Changing from a mixed to self-selected vegetarian diet - influences on blood lipids. *Journal of Human Nutrition and Dietetics* 15(5):323-9

Diabetes – When Life is too Sweet

American Diabetes Association. 2006. *American Diabetes Statistics.* www.diabetes.org and www.scientificsessions.diabetes.org

Barnard, Neal et al. 2005. The effects of a low-fat, plant-based dietary intervention on body weight, metabolism, and insulin sensitivity. *American Journal of Medicine* 118(9):991-7

Fox, Maggie. 2006. *Vegan diet reverses diabetes symptoms, study finds.* Washington (Reuters). www.lifescan.com/diabetes/news/20060727elin022/

Goff, L.M. et al. 2005. Veganism and its relationship with insulin resistance and intramyocellular lipid. *European Journal of Clinical Nutrition* 59(2):291-8

Hung, C.J. et al. 2006. Taiwanese vegetarians have higher insulin sensitivity than omnivores. *British Journal of Nutrition* 95(1):129-35

Jenkins, David J.A. et al. 2003. Type 2 diabetes and the vegetarian diet. *American Journal of Clinical Nutrition* 78(3):610S-616S

Kuo, C.S. et al. 2004. Insulin sensitivity in Chinese ovo-lactovegetarians compared with omnivores. *European Journal of Clinical Nutrition* 58(2):312-6

McCarty, M.F. 2002. Favorable Impact of a vegan diet with exercise on hemorheology: implications for control of diabetic neuropathy. *Medical Hypotheses* 58(6):476-86

Murphy, Liz. 2006. *One in three Americans born in 2000 will develop adult-onset diabetes.* American Diabetes Assoc Press release

Nicholson, Andrew S. et al. 1999. Toward Improved Management of NIDDM: A Randomized, Controlled, Pilot Intervention Using a Low-fat Vegetarian Diet. *Preventative Medicine* 29(2):87-91

Smith, Aaron. 2006. *Drug reduces vision loss in diabetics.* CNNMoney.com

Snowdon, David A. 1985. Does a Vegetarian Diet Reduce the Occurrence of Diabetes? *American Journal of Public Health* 75(5):507-512

Valachovicova, M. et al. 2005. No evidence of insulin resistance in normal weight vegetarians. A case control study. *European Journal of Nutrition* 45(1):52-4

Food Poisoning - Staying Close to the Bathroom

Donnelly, Catherine W. 2001. Listeria monocytogenes: A Continuing Challenge. *Nutrition Reviews* 59(6): 183-194

Jopp, Lou Ann. www.extension.umn.edu/extensionnews/2005/Ecoli.html   accessed 12/6/06

Krizmanic, Judy. 1995. Meat Inspection Meets the 21st Century. *Vegetarian Times* Jan 1995

Mitchell, Deborah. 2004. *Safe Foods.* New York: Signet (Penguin Books)

Quillin, Patrick. 1990. *Safe Eating.* New York: M. Evans & Co Inc.

Ryan, C.A. et al. 1987. Massive outbreak of antimicrobial-resistant salmonellosis traced to pasteurized milk. *Journal of the American Medical Association* 258(22):3269-74

Schlosser, Eric. 2001. *Fast Food Nation,* pg 9 New York: Houghton Mifflin Books

Sinclair, Upton. 1905. *The Jungle.* Pocket, 2004

Antibiotics – Penicillin Burger

American Medical Association House of Delegates. 2001. The AMA Approves Resolution to Eliminate Non-Therapeutic Use of Antibiotics in Agriculture. *Resolution 508* (A-01), May-01

Hamer, Davidson H. et al. 2002. From the Farm to the Kitchen Table: The Negative Impact of Antimicrobial Use in Animals on Humans. *Nutrition Reviews* 60(8):261-264

Sheng, Chen et al. 2004. Characterization of Multiple-Antimicrobial-Resistant Salmonella Serovars Isolated from Retail Meats. *Applied and Environmental Microbiology* 70(1):1-7

Shea, Katherine M. 2004. Nontherapeutic Use of Antimicrobial Agents in Animal Agriculture: Implications for Pediatrics. *Pediatrics* 114(3):862-868

White, David G. et al. 2001. The Isolation of Antibiotic-Resistant Salmonella from Retail Ground Meats. *New England Journal of Medicine* 345(16):1147-1154

Dementia – Losing Your Mind for the Sake of a Burger

Broxmeyer, L. 2005. Thinking the unthinkable: Alzheimer's, Creutzfeldt-Jakob and Mad Cow disease: the age-related reemergence of virulent, foodborne, bovine tuberculosis or losing your mind for the sake of a shake or burger. *Medical Hypotheses* 64(4):699-705

Cooper, J.L. 2003. Dietary lipids in the aetiology of Alzheimer's disease: implications for therapy. *Drugs & Aging* 20(6):399-418

Giem, P. et al. 1993. The incidence of dementia and intake of animal products: preliminary findings from the Adventist Health Study. *Neuroepidemiology* 12(1):28-36

Grady, Denise. 2006. Studies suggest diabetes increases Alzheimer's risk. *New York Times* July 17 2006

Kalmijn, S. et al. 1997. Dietary fat intake and the risk of incident dementia in the Rotterdam Study. *Annals of Neurology* 42(5):776-82

Luchsinger, J.A. et al. 2002. Caloric intake and the risk of Alzheimer disease. *Archives of Neurology.* 59(8):1258-63

Morris, Martha Clare et al. 2006. Associations of vegetable and fruit consumption with age-related cognitive change. *Neurology* 67:1370-1376

Morris, Martha Clare. 2004. Diet and Alzheimer's Disease: What the Evidence Shows. *Medscape General Medicine* 6(1):48

Morris, M.C. et al. 2003. Dietary fats and the risk of incident Alzheimer disease. *Archives of Neurology* 60(2):194-200

Puglielli, L. 2003. Alzheimer's disease: the cholesterol connection. *Nature Neuroscience* 6(4):345-51

Parkinson's - Steady as She Goes

Anderson, C. et al. 1999. Dietary factors in Parkinson's disease: the role of food groups and specific foods. *Movement Disorders* 14(1):21-7

de Lau, L.M. et al. 2005. Dietary fatty acids and the risk of Parkinson disease: the Rotterdam study. *Neurology* 64(12):2040-5

Logroscino, G. et al. 1996. Dietary lipids and antioxidants in Parkinson's disease: a population-based, case-control study. *Annals of Neurology* 39(1):89-94

McCarty, M.F. 2005. Does a vegan diet reduce risk for Parkinson's disease? *Medical Hypotheses* 57(3): 318-323

Park, M. et al. 2005. Consumption of milk and calcium in midlife and the future risk of Parkinson disease. *Neurology* 64(6):1047-51

Osteoporosis – Burgers and Colas May Break My Bones

Feskanich, D. et al. 1997. Milk, dietary calcium, and bone fractures in women: a 12-year prospective study. *American Journal of Public Health* 87(6):992-7

March, Alice G. et al. 1988. Vegetarian Lifestyle and bone mineral density. *American Journal of Clinical Nutrition* 48:837-41

New, Susan A. 2003. Intake of fruit and vegetables: implications for bone health. *Proceedings of the Nutrition Society* (0029-6651) 062(004):889-899

New, S.A. et al. 2000. Dietary influences on bone mass and bone metabolism: further evidence of a positive link between fruit and vegetable consumption and bone health? *American Journal of Clinical Nutrition* 71(1):142-51

New, S.A. et al. 1997. Nutritional influences on bone mineral density: a cross-sectional study in premenopausal women. *American Journal of Clinical Nutrition* 65(6):1831-9

Prynne, C.J. et al. 2006. Fruit and vegetable intakes and bone mineral status: a cross sectional study in 5 age and sex cohorts. *American Journal of Clinical Nutrition* 83(6):1420-8

Tucker, Katherine L. et al. 1999. Potassium, magnesium, and fruit and vegetable intakes are associated with greater bone mineral density in elderly men and women. *American Journal of Clinical Nutrition* 69(4): 727-736

Tylavsky, Frances A. and John J.B. Anderson. 1988. Dietary factors in bone health of elderly lactoovo-vegetarian and omnivorous women. *American Journal of Clinical Nutrition* 48:842-9

Zhang, X. et al. 2005. Prospective cohort study of soy food consumption and risk of bone fracture among post menopausal women. *Archives of Internal Medicine* 165(16):1890-5

Weinsier, Roland L. and Carlos L. Krumdieck. 2000. Dairy foods and bone health: examination of the evidence. *American Journal of Clinical Nutrition* 72(3):681-689

Arthritis – Bend Me, Stretch Me

Hafstrom, I. et al. 2001. A vegan diet free of gluten improves the signs and symptoms of rheumatoid arthritis: the effects on arthritis correlate with a reduction in antibodies to food antigens. *Rheumatology (Oxford)* 40(10):1175-9

Kjeldsen-Kragh, Jens. 1999. Rheumatoid arthritis treated with vegetarian diets. *American Journal of Clinical Nutrition* 70(3):594S-600S

Kjeldsen-Kragh, J. et al. 1994. Vegetarian diet for patients with rheumatoid arthritis--status: two years after introduction of the diet. *Clinical Rheumatology* 13(3):475-82

Kjeldsen-Kragh, J. et al. 1995. Changes in laboratory variables in rheumatoid arthritis patients during a trial of fasting and one-year vegetarian diet. *Scandinavian Journal of Rheumatology* 24(2):85-93

Kjeldsen-Kragh, J. et al. 1991. Controlled trial of fasting and one-year vegetarian diet in rheumatoid arthritis. *Lancet* 338(8772):899-902

Oliver, J.E. and A.J.Silman. 2006. Risk factors for the development of Rheumatoid Arthritis. *Scandinavian Journal of Rheumatology* 35(3):169-174

Peltonen, R. et al. 1994. Changes of faecal flora in rheumatoid arthritis during fasting and one-year vegetarian diet. *British Journal of Rheumatology* 33(7):638-43

Toivanen, P. and E. Eerola. 2002. A vegan diet changes the intestinal flora. *Rheumatology* 41:950-951

Triolo, G. et al. 2002. Humoral and cell mediated immune response to cow's milk proteins in Behçet's disease. *Annals of the Rheumatic Diseases* 61:459-462

Gallstones and Kidney Stones – Ouch!

Chung-Jyi, Tsai et al. 2004. Frequent nut consumption and decreased risk of cholecystectomy in women. *American Journal of Clinical Nutrition* 80(1):76-81

Chung-Jyi, Tsai et al. 2004. Dietary Protein and the Risk of Cholecystectomy in a Cohort of US Women. *American Journal of Epidemiology* 160:11-18

Curhan, G.C. et al. 2004. Dietary factors and the risk of incident kidney stones in younger women: Nurses' Health Study II. *Archives of Internal Medicine* 164(8):885-91

Giovanni, Misciagna et al. 1999. Diet, physical activity, and gallstones—a population-based, case-control study in southern Italy. *American Journal of Clinical Nutrition* 69(1):120-126

Pixley, F. and J. Mann. 1988. Dietary factors in the aetiology of gall stones: a case control study.,*Gut* 29(11):1511-5

Pixley, F. et al. 1985. Effect of vegetarianism on development of gall stones in women. *British Medical Journal (Clin Res Ed)* 291(6487):11-2

Remer, T. and F. Manz, 1994. Estimation of the renal net acid excretion by adults consuming diets containing variable amounts of protein. *American Journal of Clinical Nutrition* 59(6):1356-61

Robertson, W.G. 1987. Diet and calcium stones. *Mineral and Electrolyte Metabolism* 13(4):228-34

Robertson, W.G. et al. 1982. Prevalence of urinary stone disease in vegetarians. *European Urology*. 8(6):334-9

Robertson, W.G. et al. 1979. Should recurrent calcium oxalate stone formers become vegetarians? *British Journal of Urology* 51(6):427-31

Siener, R. and A. Hesse. 2003. The effect of a vegetarian and different omnivorous diets on urinary risk factors for uric acid stone formation. *European Journal of Nutrition* 42(6):332-7

Straub, M. and R.E. Hautmann. 2005. Developments in stone prevention. *Current Opinion in Urology* 15(2):119-26

Wahl, C. and B. Hess. 2000. Kidney calculi--is nutrition a trigger or treatment? *Therapeutica Umschau* 57(3):138-45

Being Up Front About Our Rear Ends

National Center for Health Statistics. 2002. Dietary Intake of Macronutrients, Micronutrients, and Other Dietary Constituents: United States, 1988–94. *Vital and Health Statistics* 11(245)

Adamidis, D. et al. 2000. Fiber intake and childhood appendicitis. *International Journal of Food Sciences & Nutrition* 51(3):153-7

Alonso-Coello, P. et al. 2006. Fiber for the treatment of hemorrhoids complications: a systematic review and meta-analysis. *American Journal of Gastroenterology* 101(1):181-8

Arnbjornsson, E. 1983. Acute appendicitis and dietary fiber. *Archives of Surgery* 118(7):868-70

Black, J. 2002. Acute appendicitis in Japanese soldiers in Burma: support for the "fibre" theory. *Gut* 51:297

Burkitt, Dennis. 1979. *Eat Right*. New York: Arco Publishing

Floch, M.H. and I. Bina. 2004. The natural history of diverticulitis: fact and theory. *Journal of Clinical Gastroenterology* 38(5 Suppl):S2-7

Gear, J.S. et al. 1979. Symptomless diverticular disease and intake of dietary fibre. *Lancet.* 1(8115):511-4

Gray, D.S. 1995. The clinical uses of dietary fiber. *American Family Physician.* 51(2):419-26

Handler, S. 1983. Dietary fiber: Can it prevent certain colonic diseases? *Postgraduate Medicine* 73(2):301-7

Kang, J.Y., D. Melville and J.D. Maxwell. 2004. Epidemiology and management of diverticular disease of the colon. *Drugs & Aging* 21(4):211-28

Kitoraga, N.F. and V.V. Mishchenko. 1995. The prevention of hemorrhoids in sailors. *Likars'ka Sprava* (9-12):179-81

Marlett, J.A. et al. 2002. Position of the American Dietetic Association: health implications of dietary fiber. *Journal of the American Dietetic Association* 102(7):993-1000

Mimura, T. et al. 2002. Pathophysiology of diverticular disease. *Best Practice & Research Clinical Gastroenterology* 16(4):563-76

Nair, P. and J.F. Mayberry. 1994. Vegetarianism, dietary fibre and gastro-intestinal disease. *Digestive Diseases* 12(3):177-85

Ozick, L.A. et al. 1994. Pathogenesis, diagnosis, and treatment of diverticular disease of the colon. *Gastroenterologist* 2(4):299-310

Parra-Blanco, A. 2006. Colonic diverticular disease: pathophysiology and clinical picture. *Digestion* 73 Suppl 1:47-57

Painter, N.S. 1982. Diverticular disease of the colon. The first of the Western diseases shown to be due to a deficiency of dietary fibre. *South African Medical Journal* 61(26):1016-20

Sanjoaquin, M.A. et al. 2004. Nutrition and lifestyle in relation to bowel movement frequency: a cross-sectional study of 20630 men and women in EPIC-Oxford. *Public Health Nutrition* 7(1):77-83

Vanderpool, D.M. 1986. Dietary fiber: its role in preventing gastrointestinal disease. *Southern Medical Journal* 79(10):1201-4

West, A.B. and M. Losada. 2004. The pathology of diverticulosis coli. *Journal of Clinical Gastroenterology* 38(5 Suppl):S11-6

Editorial. 2000. How to treat hemorrhoids. *British Medical Journal* 321:582-583

Why Didn't My Doctor Tell Me?

Williams, C.L., M. Bollella and E. Wynder. 1994. Preventive cardiology in primary care. *Atherosclerosis* 108 Suppl:S117-26

Wood, D. 1999. Guidelines--a missed opportunity. *Atherosclerosis* 143 Suppl 1:S7-12

What Am I to Believe?

Amsterdam, Ezra A. 2006. The Low-Fat Diet that "wasn't." *Preventive Cardiology* 9(2):121

Chapter 5 - Global Hunger

Altschul, Aaron. 1965. Proteins: *Their Chemistry and Politics.* pg 265. New York: Basic Books

Brown, Lester R. 1994. *Facing Food Scarcity.* Washington D.C.: Worldwatch Institute

Brown, Lester R. 1995. *Who Will Feed China?* pgs 98,115,126,139. New York: W.W. Norton & Company

Brown, Lester. 1999. *The United States and China, The Soybean Connection.* Washington D.C.: Worldwatch Institute press notice, 9 November

Diamond, Harvey. 1990. *Your Heart Your Planet.* Santa Monica CA: Hay House, Inc.

Homer-Dixon,Thomas. 1993. *Environmental Scarcity and Global Security,* pg 25. Foreign Policy Association

Kindall, Henry W and David Pimentel. 1994. Constraints on the Expansion Of The Global Food Supply. *Ambio* 23(3) The Royal Swedish Academy of Sciences

Nierenberg, Danielle. 2005. *Happier Meals.* Washington D.C.: World Watch Paper 171

Phillipson, John. 1966. *Ecological Energetics.* Edward Arnold (Publishers) Ltd

Pimentel, D. 2002. *Feeding the World.* Broadcast on 7/20/2002 Australian Broadcasting Company.

Pimentel, D. 2004. *Livestock production and Energy Use.* Cleveland C. ed. Encyclopedia of Energy. Elsevier

Pimentel, D. et al. 1997. Water Usage Source. *Bioscience* 42: 97-106

Platt McGinn, Anne. 1998. *Rocking the Boat: Conserving Fisheries and Protecting Jobs.* Washington D.C.: World Watch Institute

Scharffenberg, John A. 1979. *Problems with Meat,* pgs 65, 67. Santa Barbara CA: Woodbridge Press Publishing Company

United Nations- Food and Agriculture Organization. 2006. *Livestock, Environment and Development Initiative.* FAO Agriculture 21. www.virtualcentre.org/en/frame.htm

United Nations-Food and Agriculture Organization. 2004. FAOSTAT Statistical Database 12/20/2004

USDA Agricultural Statistics. 1984. www.usda.gov/nass/pubs/agr4all.pdf

World Health Organization (WHO). 2002. Diet, nutrition and the prevention of chronic diseases. *Draft report of the joint WHO/ FAO expert consultation.* April

Worldwatch Institute. 1998.*United States Leads World Meat Stampede.* Press release, 2 July

Wynne-Tyson, Jon. 1979. *Food for a Future.* New York: Universe Books

Chapter 6 - The Environmental Crisis

Browner, Carol M. 2001. *Environmental assessment of proposed revisions to the National Pollutant Discharge Elimination System regulation and effluent limitations guidelines for concentrated animal feeding operations.* Washington, D.C.: Engineering and Analysis Division, Office of Science and Technology, U.S. Environmental Protection Agency

Burkholder, JoAnn M. et al. 1997. Impacts to a Coastal River and Estuary from Rupture of a Large Swine Waste Holding Lagoon. *Journal of Environmental Quality* 26(6):1451-66

Detenbeck, N.E. et al. 2000. A test of watershed classification systems for ecological risk assessment. *Environmental Toxicology & Chemistry* 19:1174-1181 Pensacola, FL: SETAC Press

Diamond, Harvey. 1990. *Your Heart Your Planet.* Santa Monica CA: Hay House, Inc.

Eshel, Gidon and Pamela Martin. 2006. *Vegan Diets Healthier for Planet, People than Meat Diets.* www.medicalnewstoday.com/medicalnews.php?newsid=41660

Eshel, Gidon and Pamela Martin. 2006. Diet, Energy and Global Warming. *Earth Interactions* 10(9):15

Leitzmann, Claus. 2003. Nutrition ecology: the contribution of vegetarian diets. *American Journal of Clinical Nutrition* 78(3): 657S-659S

Mallin, Michael. 2000. Impacts of industrial animal agriculture on Rivers and Estuaries. *American Scientist* 88(1):26

Miller, G. Tyler. 1993. *Living in the Environment, Eighth Edition.* pg 365. Belmont, CA: Wadsworth Publishing Company

Moran, Joseph M., Michael D. Morgan and James H. Wiersma. 1986. *Introduction to Environmental Science, Second Edition,* pg 573. San Francisco, CA: W.H. Freeman and Company

Nierenberg, Diane. 2005. *Happier Meals* pgs 30,58. Washington D.C.: World Watch Institute

Pimentel, David and Marcia Pimentel. 2003. Sustainability of meat-based and plant-based diets and the environment. *American Journal of Clinical Nutrition* 78(3):660S-663S

Pimentel, D. 1979. Food Calories produced per calorie input from fossil fuel. *Food, Energy and Society* pg 56-59. New York: John Wiley and Sons

Pimentel, D. 2004. *Livestock Production and Energy Use.* Cleveland C. ed. Encyclopedia of Energy. Elsevier

Pimentel, D. 2003. World population, food, natural resources and survival. *World Futures* 59(3-4):145-67

Reijnders, Lucas and Sam Soret. 2003. Quantification of the environmental impact of different dietary protein choices. *American Journal of Clinical Nutrition* 78(3):664S-668S

United States Department of Agriculture, Economic Research Service. 1991. *World Agricultural Supply and Demand Estimates,* WASDE-256, tables 256-6, 256-7, 256-16, 256-19, and 256-23. Washington, D.C.: USDA

Weiss, Kenneth. 2002. Salmon Farms are Factory Farms: Dioxins, Pollution and Environmental Carelessness. *Los Angeles Times,* Dec 9. www.organicconsumers.org/irrad/salmonfarms.cfm

Zaslowsky Dyan, 1989. A Public Beef: Are Grazing Cattle Turning The American West Into a New Desert? *Harrowsmith Country Life.* Laval, QC, Canada: Malcolm Publishing Inc.

Chapter 7 - Saving the Animals with Every Bite

Bentham, Jeremy. 1789. *An Introduction to the Principles of Morals and Legislation.* Oxford: Clarendon Press

Byrd, Senator Robert. 2001. Congressional Record July 9

Chervova, L.S. 1997. Pain sensitivity and behaviour of fish [original title: Bolevaya chuvstvitel'nost' i povedenie ryb]. Voprosy Ikhtiologii. 37(1): 106-111

Franklin, Benjamin.1996. *Autobiography.* New York: Dover Publications

Goodall, Jane. 2005. *Harvest for Hope.* Time Warner Book Group

Masci, David. 1996. Fighting over animal rights. *Congressional Quarterly* Aug 2

Paine, Thomas. 2006. *The Age of Reason.* New York:Citadel (New Ed Edition)

Penn, William. 1792. *Some Fruits of Solitude.* Friends United Press

Scully, Matthew. 2002. *Dominion: The Power of Man, the Suffering of Animals, and the Call to Mercy.* pgs 101, 290. New York: St. Martin's Press

Chapter 8 – Food and Faith

Berlin, Adele Ed. 2003. *The Jewish Study Bible: featuring The Jewish Publication Society TANAKH Translation*. Oxford University Press, USA

Berman, Louis A. 1982. *Vegetarianism and the Jewish Tradition*. New York: KTAV Publishing House Inc.

Gregerson, Jon. 1994. *Vegetarianism. A History*. Fremont CA: Jain Publishing Co.

Kalechofsky, Roberta. 1995. *Rabbis and Vegetarianism: An Evolving Tradition*. Micah Publications

Kalechofsky Roberta. 1998. *Vegetarian Judaism*. Micah Publications

Kapleau Roshi, Philip. 1982. *To Cherish All Life*. San Francisco: Harper & Row

Rosen, Steven. 1987. *Food for the Spirit*. New York: Bala Books

Schwartz, Richard H. 1988. *Judaism and Vegetarianism*. Micah Publications

Talmud. Chulin 84a

The Holy Scriptures. Genesis 1:29, 1:30. Proverbs 12:10. Psalms 145:9. Isaiah 11:6, 11:7. Hosea 2:20. Daniel 1:11 - 1:16. 1955. Philadelphia: The Jewish Publication Society of America

Wansbrough, Henry ed. 1985. *The New Jerusalem Bible*. New York: Doubleday

White, Ellen G. 1976. *Counsels on Diet and Foods*. Hagerstown MD: Review & Herald Publishing Assoc.

White, E.G. 1982. *Health and Happiness*. Phoenix AZ: Inspiration Books

Suggested Reading

General Interest Books

Akers, Keith. 1989. *A Vegetarian Source Book*. Denver, CO: Vegetarian Press

Barnard, Neal. 1995. *Eat Right Live Longer*. Three Rivers Press.

Barnard, Neal. 2007. *Dr. Neal Barnard's Program for Reversing Diabetes: The Scientifically Proven System for Reversing Diabetes Without Drugs*. Rodale

Berman, Louis A. 1982. *Vegetarianism and the Jewish Tradition*. New York: KTAV Publishing House Inc.

Brown, Lester R. 1995. *Who Will Feed China? Wake up call for a small planet*. New York: W.W. Norton & Company

Campbell, T. Colin. 2004. *The China Study*. Dallas, TX: Benbella Books

Cox, Peter. 2002. *You Don't Need Meat*. New York: St. Martin's Press

Diamond, Harvey. 1990. *Your Heart Your Planet*. Santa Monica, CA: Hay House, Inc.

Ferber, Elizabeth. 1998. *The Vegetarian Life: How to be a Veggie in a Meat-Eating World*. New York: Berkley Books

Foster, Ray L and Frances L. 2003. *The Veggie Book: The "How to" Book for Beginner Vegetarians*. Newstart Healthcare.

Fuhrman, Joel. 2003. *Eat to Live*. New York: Little, Brown and Company.

Giehl, Dudley. 1979. *Vegetarianism: A Way of Life*. New York: Harper and Row

Goodall, Jane. 2005. *Harvest for Hope: A guide for mindful eating*. Time Warner Book Group

Gregerson, Jon. 1994. *Vegetarianism. A History*. Fremont, CA: Jain Publishing Co.

Iacobbo, Karen and Michael. 2006. *Vegetarians and Vegans in America Today*. Westport, CT: Praeger

Iacobbo, Karen and Michael. 2004. *Vegetarian America*. Westport, CT: Praeger

International Society for Krishna Consciousness. 1991. *The Higher Taste: A Guide to Gourmet Vegetarian Cooking and Karma Free Diet*. The Bhaktivedanta Book Trust.

Joyce, Marilyn. 1995. *5 Minutes to Health*. Vibrant Health Academy

Kapleau Roshi, Philip. 1982. *To Cherish All Life*. San Francisco, CA: Harper & Row

Kushi, Michio. 1987. *Crime and Diet*. New York: Japan Publications

McDougall, John A. 1983. *The McDougall Plan*. Piscataway, NJ: New Century Publishers Inc.

McDougall, John. 2006. *Dr. McDougall's Digestive Tune Up*. Summertown, TN: The Book Publishing Company

Melina, Vesanto and Brenda Davis. 2000. *Becoming Vegan*. Summertown, TN: The Book Publishing Company

Messina, Virginia and Mark Messina. 1996. *The Vegetarian Way*. New York: Three Rivers Press

Messina, Mark and Virgina Messina. 1996. *The Dietitian's Guide to Vegetarian Diets*. Gaithersburg, MD: Aspen Publishers

Moore, Shirley T. and Mary P. Byers. 1978. *A Vegetarian Diet, What it is; How to make it Healthful and Enjoyable.* Santa Barbara, CA: Woodbridge Press

Nedley, Neil. 1999. *Proof Positive: How to Reliably Combat Disease and Achieve Optimal Health Through Nutrition and Lifestyle.* Ardmore, OK.

Nierenberg, Danielle. 2005. *Happier Meals: Rethinking the global meat industry.* Washington D.C.: World Watch Paper 171

Ornish, Dean. 1996. *Dr Dean Ornish's Program for Reversing Heart Disease.* New York: Ivy Books.

Ornish, Dean. 2001. *Eat More Weigh Less.* New York: Harper Collins Publishers

Physicians Committee for Responsible Medicine. 2002. *Healthy Eating for Life for Children.* New York: John Wiley & Sons

Rice, Pamela. 2005. *101 Reasons Why I'm a Vegetarian.* New York: Lantern Books

Robbins, John. 1987. *Diet for a New America.* Walpole, NH: Stillpoint Publishing

Rosen, Steven. 1997. *Diet For Transcendence.* Badger, CA: Torchlight Publishing

Rudd, Geoffrey L. 1956. *Why Kill for Food?* Wilmslow Cheshire, UK: The Vegetarian Society

Scharffenberg, John A. 1979. *Problems with Meat.* Santa Barbara, CA: Woodbridge Press Publishing Company

Schlosser, Eric. 2001. *Fast Food Nation.* New York: Houghton Mifflin Books

Schwartz, Richard H. 1988. *Judaism and Vegetarianism.* Micah Publications

Scully, Matthew. 2002. *Dominion: The Power of Man, the suffering of animals, and the call to mercy.* New York: St. Martin's Press

Vegetarians of Washington. 2004. *Veg-Feasting in the Pacific Northwest.* Summertown, TN: The Book Publishing Company

White, Ellen G. 1976. *Counsels on Diet and Foods.* Hagerstown MD: Review & Herald Publishing Assoc.

White, E.G. 1982. *Health and Happiness.* Phoenix AZ: Inspiration Books

Wynne-Tyson, Jon. 1979. *Food for a Future.* New York: Universe Books

Cookbooks

Allen, Zell. 2006. *The Nut Gourmet.* Summertown, TN: The Book Publishing Company

Bloomfield, Barb. *More Fabulous Beans.* Summertown, TN: The Book Publishing Company

Burton, Dreena. 2001. *The Everyday Vegan.* Vancouver, BC: Arsenal Pulp Press

Gartenstein, Devra. 2000. *The Accidental Vegan.* Freedom, CA: The Crossing Press

Geier, Catherine and Carol Brown. 2005. *The Café Flora Cookbook.* New York: The Berkley Publishing Group

Grogan, Bryanna Clark. 2000. *Authentic Chinese Cuisine.* Summertown, TN: The Book Publishing Company

Hagler, Louise. 1998. *Tofu and Soyfoods Cookery.* Summertown, TN: The Book Publishing Company

Lair, Cynthia. 1997. *Feeding the Whole Family*. Seattle, WA: Moonsmile Press

Petrovna, Tanya. 2003. *The Native Foods Restaurant Cookbook*. Shambhala

Reseck, Heather. 2002. *Fix-It-Fast*. Hagerstown, MD: Review and Herald Publishing

Robertson, Robin. 1996. *366 Healthful Ways to Cook Tofu and other Meat Alternatives*. Plume (Penguin Books)

Shastri, Sunita K. *Indian Vegetarian Delights*

Stepaniak, Joanne. 1994. *The Uncheese Cookbook*. Summertown, TN: The Book Publishing Company

Vegetarians of Washington. 2005. *The Veg-Feasting Cookbook*. Summertown, TN: The Book Publishing Company

Index of Tables and Illustrations

(Continued)

Index

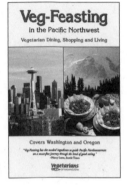
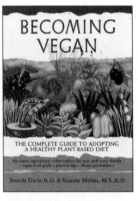
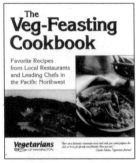
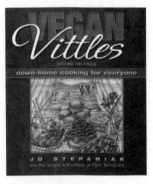
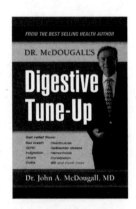